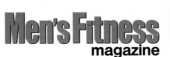

COMPLETE GUIDE TO
HOME WORKOUTS

By Jon Lipsey

Design Ian Jackson
Subeditor Michael Donlevy
Photography Tom Miles
Model Tom Dyer@WAthletic

Thanks to Escape Fitness
and Fitness Superstore

For more information on Men's Fitness magazine, go to **www.mensfitnessmagazine.co.uk**
To subscribe call **0844 844 0081**

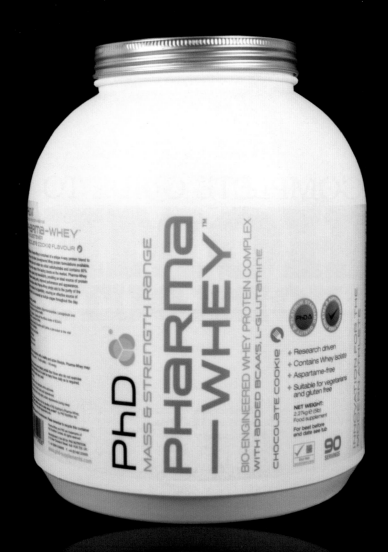
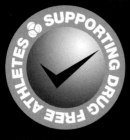

Contents

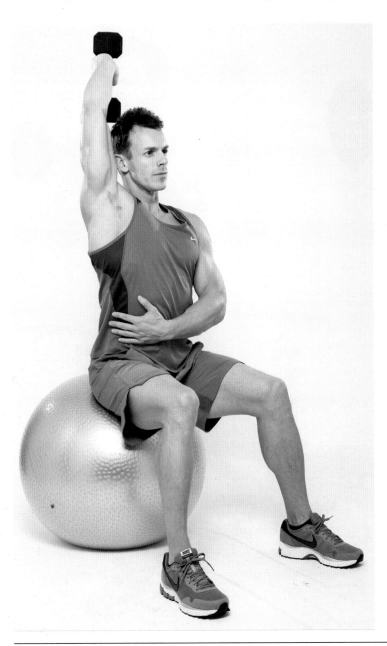

Contents

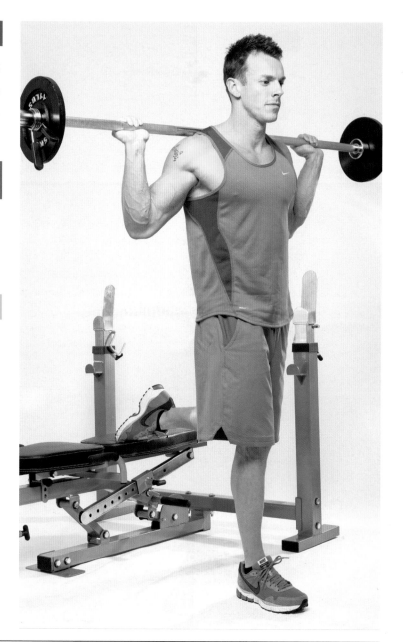

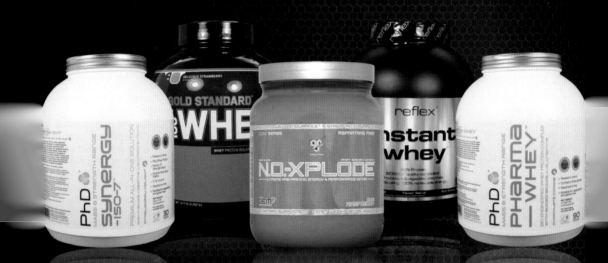

Getting started **I** Introduction

Training begins now

Working out at home is an accessible way of getting fitter and stronger. This book tells you everything you need to know to hit your muscle targets

Welcome to the *Men's Fitness Complete Guide To Home Workouts*, a comprehensive training resource for anyone who wants to exercise at home. By using the exercises, advice and workouts in this book, you'll develop a lean and muscular physique. The moves and training systems we've selected will give you great results whether you've been working out for years or are a complete beginner. All you have to do is make sure that you structure your workouts to give your muscles progressively tougher training challenges.

Working out at home is incredibly accessible because you can start without having to buy any kit. If you want to make fantastic progress, buying simple equipment such as dumb-bells and a gym ball will allow you to do a wide variety of workouts, helping you to keep progressing and stay motivated.

What's in the guide?

The book starts with a clear and full guide to basic training theory. By understanding the key variables involved in a workout, such as the number of sets and reps you perform, you stand a better chance of achieving the body you've always wanted.

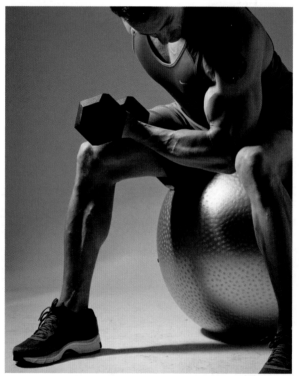

The exercise demonstration and workout pages of the book are split up into chapters involving different bits of kit. The first contains all the best moves you can do by using bodyweight alone, as well as some sample workouts you can use depending on what you want to get out of your training sessions. That's followed by a chapter on dumb-bells and gym balls, which includes a gear guide, 65 muscle-building moves and 15 sample workouts. The Extra Kit chapter explores how adding a few simple items such as a pull-up bar, medicine ball and resistance band can allow you to train in new and productive ways. The barbell and bench chapter completes the training section

and shows you how to use big moves for maximum muscle growth.

If you're really serious about building a home gym, you may want to invest in a cardio machine or a multigym. The home gym machine section will tell you what qualities you should be looking for so you make the right purchase.

What you eat has as much of an impact on your body shape as the amount of training you do. That's why we've included a chapter that gives you clear advice about how to eat healthily, where fresh food is in and gimmicky diet plans are off the menu. There's also a sample meal plan and a thorough guide to sports supplements.

How to use this book

You can use the *Complete Guide To Home Workouts* whether you're a beginner or an experienced exerciser. The kit guide sections give you advice on how to buy home workout kit. The exercise demonstration pages show you how to perform effective moves with perfect form while the workout pages give you examples of common training methods. You can then design your own workouts by arranging the exercises according to the principles of your chosen training method.

Muscle myths
Don't let these common muscle myths hamper your training

Myth: Weight training will make you bulky
Reality: Even if you train regularly and push yourself to your limit, you won't suddenly sprout huge muscles. Training properly will increase your muscle size but this happens over time and, if you don't want your workouts to have a muscle-building effect, you need to adjust key variables, such as how many reps you perform, so they have more of either a strength or endurance effect than a muscle gain one.

Myth: Endless crunches will give you a six-pack
Reality: Doing crunches will strengthen and define your abs but it will do little to remove any body fat that's hiding them. You can't lose fat from any one part of your body so, if you want to shift your spare tyre, eat healthily

and perform exercises that burn lots of calories. Crunches burn comparatively few calories, so they're not good for getting rid of your gut. And doing hundreds of any exercise is an inefficient way of training because if you can do that many reps the movement isn't challenging enough to stimulate new muscle growth.

Myth: Running is better for fat loss than lifting weights
Reality: Intense weights sessions will burn plenty of calories and have a fat-loss effect. High-intensity circuits give you the benefit of an aerobic workout, which improves your heart and lung function, as well as strengthen muscles. Running is good for developing your heart and lungs but won't build much muscle.

Myth: It's safer to lift weights slowly
Reality: In rehabilitation, patients are told to perform exercises at a slow tempo to retrain their bodies to execute movement smoothly, a tactic that has crept into gyms. But as long as you're always in control of the lifting and lowering phases of an exercise you won't set yourself up for an injury. Indeed, performing reps with speed trains the muscles to react quickly in unexpected, real-world situations, which is how you really protect yourself from injury. It also activates more muscle fibres, leading to greater gains.

Myth: Machines are safer than freeweights
Reality: The makers of weights machines advertise that their equipment isolates

target muscles and prevents injury by eliminating room for error. But the restrictive movements of machines might actually increase the risk of injury. Machines are fixed and rigid and therefore limit natural movement, whereas when you use freeweights your body naturally makes adjustments throughout the exercise's range of motion according to your strength level, speed of movement, and proficiency.

Myth: More training means more muscle
Reality: Muscle growth happens while you're recovering, not while you're working out. If you don't leave enough time between sessions, you won't let your muscles complete the repair process that makes them bigger and stronger.

Advice for beginners
If you're new to weight training, follow this advice to avoid injury

■ **Warm up properly**
Always warm up properly before doing any serious exercise (see p20). This will help you to stay injury free.

■ **Stop if it hurts**
If you feel pain at any time during your workout, stop immediately. The saying 'no pain, no gain' is popular in with old-school PE teachers who don't know what they're talking about. Working through pain could do serious damage to muscles, joints or tendons.

■ **Watch your form**
Maintain perfect form for every repetition of

every exercise. Each exercise in this book comes with detailed notes on form. If you don't have good form you won't get the full benefit of the exercise and may injure yourself.

■ **Start light**
Pick a weight you can manage easily the first time you perform any lifting exercise. This way you can concentrate on performing the exercise perfectly, and then you can build up the weight over time.

■ **Brace your core**
You can help to stabilise your body and reduce your injury risk by engaging your

core during an exercise. To do this, start by ensuring that you are standing or sitting up straight with your hips in line with your torso. Now imagine that someone is about to punch you in the stomach and you have to tense your abdominal muscles to take the blow. You need to maintain that contraction throughout the move to protect your lower back from muscle strains.

■ **Keep training**
For more advice on training, plus detailed workouts and eating plans, see *Men's Fitness* magazine every month. Go to mensfitnessmagazine.co.uk for more details.

Getting started I Introduction

Home vs Gym

Working out at home and working out in a gym both have advantages and disadvantages. Here's how to get the most out of a home set-up

One of the best things about working out at home is that it's accessible. In fact, you could start right now, even if you don't have any kit. That's because you can do lots of challenging exercises, such as press-ups and chair dips, just by using your bodyweight. You can't do everything with bodyweight alone but the good news is that you don't need lots of kit to lose fat and build muscle. A gym ball and a set of dumb-bells will allow

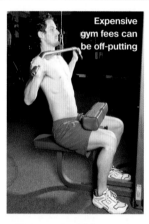

Expensive gym fees can be off-putting

you to perform a wide variety of exercises. Adding a couple of accessories such as a medicine ball and a pull-up bar will further increase your options. Finally, a barbell and bench will let you lift heavy weights for real strength and size gains. If you're really serious about fitness you can add a squat rack and cardio machines but if you're starting out, the simple and cost-effective kit in the workout chapters of this book can whip you into excellent shape.

Find your space

Before you start, make sure you have enough space to exercise without damaging either yourself or a priceless family heirloom. A seven-foot by seven-foot space should just about be enough. Choosing a room with a high-ish ceiling is also advisable, if you want to avoid cracking your head or hands during jumping moves. And wherever you work out, don't compromise form if you're tight for space.

Home gym advantages

✓ It's cost effective
You can do a huge variety of moves with a gym ball, dumb-bells and a pull-up bar, the combined cost of which can be under £50. The more kit you buy the more expensive it'll be but you can build a versatile home gym without breaking the bank. If you stick to your plans and achieve your fitness goals, you'll be glad you made the investment.

✓ You'll save time
A major benefit of working out at home is that you don't have to travel if you want to train.

✓ It's flexible
Your home gym will always be open so if you suddenly get

the urge to do a workout, you can. And if you want to train at anti-social hours, you can do that too.

✓ You don't have to queue for kit
Unless you invite friends to join you, you'll be the only one using your kit. That means no waiting around for someone else to finish their sets and you can make sure you stick to your rest periods.

✓ No gym villains
In your own home you won't have to contend with posers on mobile phones, people with hygiene issues and ugly naked men who spend far too long towelling themselves off in the changing rooms.

The drawbacks
If you're very short of space, you may find working out at home difficult. But provided you have the space, there isn't much you can't do with the kit included in this book. There are, however, some bits of kit you'd find in a commercial gym that can enhance your workouts. If you don't have a squat rack (a stand that holds a barbell so you don't have to lift it off the ground every time you want to perform a lift), for example, you'll find it hard to do heavy squats and bench presses.

Another advantage commercial gyms have over home set-ups is the support network. A good personal trainer can work out a programme tailored to your goals,

record your progression and give you advice and motivation when you need it. Gym staff are also on hand to offer technique advice if you're unsure how to perform a lift. Follow the comprehensive form guides that accompany every exercise in this book, though, and you'll be demonstrating perfect form.

Unless you're prepared to spend serious cash, your home gym won't have the variety of cardio machines offered by commercial gyms. But this doesn't have to hamper your fitness. Running outside can give you great cardiovascular workouts, as can performing weights circuits where you do exercises back to back with light weights.

Introduction | Getting started

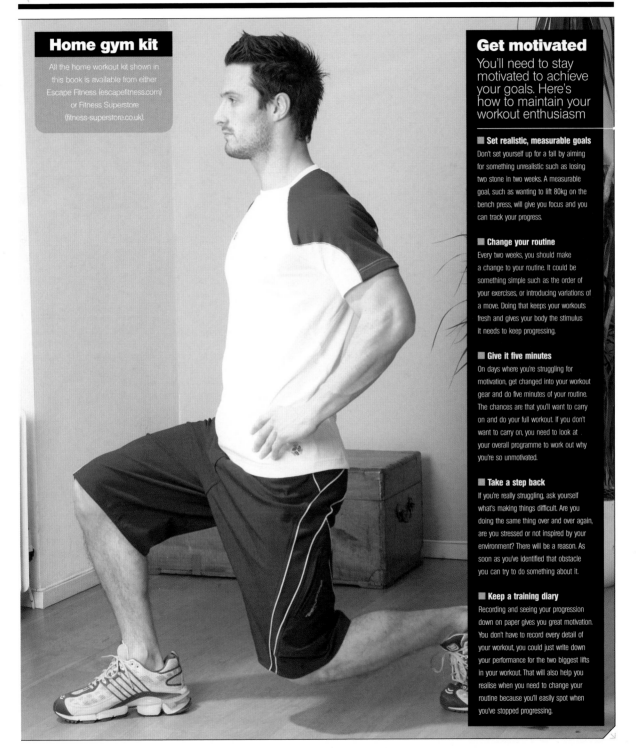

Home gym kit

All the home workout kit shown in this book is available from either Escape Fitness (escapefitness.com) or Fitness Superstore (fitness-superstore.co.uk).

Get motivated

You'll need to stay motivated to achieve your goals. Here's how to maintain your workout enthusiasm

■ Set realistic, measurable goals

Don't set yourself up for a fall by aiming for something unrealistic such as losing two stone in two weeks. A measurable goal, such as wanting to lift 80kg on the bench press, will give you focus and you can track your progress.

■ Change your routine

Every two weeks, you should make a change to your routine. It could be something simple such as the order of your exercises, or introducing variations of a move. Doing that keeps your workouts fresh and gives your body the stimulus it needs to keep progressing.

■ Give it five minutes

On days where you're struggling for motivation, get changed into your workout gear and do five minutes of your routine. The chances are that you'll want to carry on and do your full workout. If you don't want to carry on, you need to look at your overall programme to work out why you're so unmotivated.

■ Take a step back

If you're really struggling, ask yourself what's making things difficult. Are you doing the same thing over and over again, are you stressed or not inspired by your environment? There will be a reason. As soon as you've identified that obstacle you can try to do something about it.

■ Keep a training diary

Recording and seeing your progression down on paper gives you great motivation. You don't have to record every detail of your workout, you could just write down your performance for the two biggest lifts in your workout. That will also help you realise when you need to change your routine because you'll easily spot when you've stopped progressing.

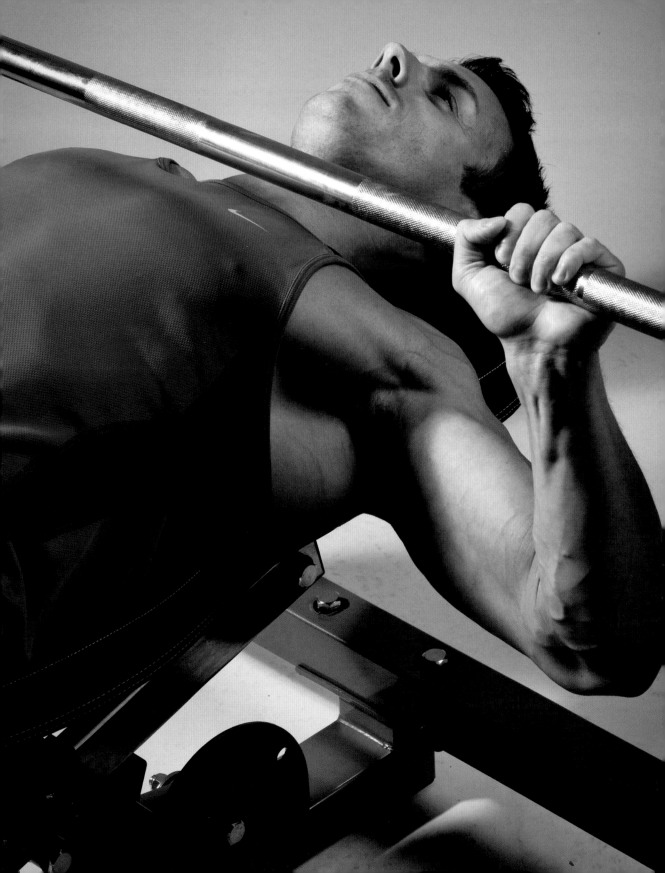

Designing your workouts

Use the following advice to create workouts that will help you achieve your exercise goals

Starting a workout without knowing what you want to achieve, what exercises you're going to do or how you're going to perform them isn't going to give you optimum results. To achieve your workout aims, you need to design and stick to a specific programme. But you can't do that without understanding the key variables involved in how you perform each exercise and how you design your workouts. The main variables to think about are:

■ **Repetitions**
Also known as reps, this is the number of times you lift a weight or perform a particular exercise within a set.

■ **Sets**
Groups of repetitions performed back to back.

■ **Rest**
The inactive time you take between sets and exercises.

■ **Tempo**
The speed at which reps are performed.

■ **Frequency**
This refers to how often you perform a workout.

Once you understand these variables, you can decide how to use them to achieve your muscle-building goals. There is, however, no such thing as the perfect muscle-building routine. To understand that, you need to have a basic appreciation of what makes your muscles grow. When you perform resistance exercises you create microscopic tears in your muscles. Your body then responds to this stimulus and your muscles repair themselves to become bigger and stronger than they were before. But if you continue to repeat the same workout your body will stop adapting to the stimulus and your gains will plateau. To avoid that happening, you need to make sure you regularly alter the variables described above.

The exercises you choose to perform and the order in which you perform them will also have an effect on the results you see. This section will give you all the information you need to decide what reps, sets, rest and tempo to use as well as a brief guide on how to order exercises.

The most common and effective methods of grouping exercises have been given workout names. These names tell you broadly what

the session involves so, for example, a 'superset' workout will typically involve doing pairs of exercises performed back to back, resting between sets of pairs of exercises rather than sets of individual exercises. More information about these common routines can be found in the workouts section of each kit chapter as you progress through the rest of the book.

It's worth noting that the following advice is a guide and that there isn't one

The number of repetitions you perform of each exercise is the most important workout variable

perfect way of addressing workout variables. That's partly because people respond to training in slightly different ways and partly because strength and conditioning research is constantly evolving. But it's still rare that new findings challenge fundamental workout principles and the reason that conventions, such as performing multiple sets rather than single sets, exist is because there's substantial and credible sports science to back them up.

Repetitions
The number of repetitions per set you perform of each exercise is, arguably, the most important workout variable. The reps you choose to perform will affect all the other variables and they have a huge impact on whether the primary effect of your workout is developing muscle strength, size or endurance.

Strength coaches generally agree that certain repetition ranges have particular training effects and these are shown

in the box on page 14. Low reps in the 1-8 range are best for building strength; between 8-12 reps is best for adding muscle mass and 12-20 reps will develop muscle endurance. These are, however, broad guides and are on a spectrum rather than self-contained blocks. Performing three or seven repetitions of an exercise, for example, will have a strength building effect but the seven repetitions will have more of a size development effect than performing three repetitions

Getting started **I** Training principles

because it's closer to the size gain range of the spectrum.

In each case, to get the desired effect, you should aim to reach failure (the point where you are unable to complete another rep without compromising perfect form) at your target rep count on the final set of the exercise. If you reach your target rep and feel that you could perform more reps, you're not using a heavy enough weight.

It's also important to remember that these rep ranges are general guides. Not everyone responds to resistance training in exactly the same way and even different muscles in the body can respond differently, depending on their function. Slow-twitch muscle fibres (the smaller muscle fibres involved in long-distance endurance efforts), for example, will generally experience strength gains at a higher rep range than fast-twitch muscle fibres (the larger fibres involved in short, explosive movements).

Your level of training experience will also play a part in the results you see. Generally, people new to weight training will develop strength into a slightly higher rep range than more experienced exercisers.

Sets

The convention for standard weight training programmes

Aim to reach failure – where you are unable to complete another rep without perfect form

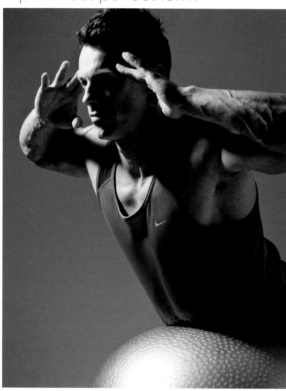

is to recommend doing 3 sets of 10-12 repetitions because that allows you to fatigue your muscles in a time that will maximise your training effect. Current guidelines from the American College

Of Sports Medicine (ACSM), for example, advise beginners to do between 1-3 sets of 8-12 repetitions.

The number of sets you perform should be directly linked to the number of

repetitions you do. Generally, the two should be inversely related so the more sets you do, the fewer reps you should perform and vice versa.

Studies have shown that the most effective workout duration for strength and muscle building is about 45 minutes. After that, your training efforts can be counterproductive, because testosterone levels drop and stress hormone levels rise, so the number of exercises in your workout should affect how many sets you perform. If you include a high number of exercises in your workout you may need to reduce the sets per exercise you perform.

Your level of experience should also be a factor. If you're very new to training, you may want to consider doing one or two sets of each exercise to get your muscles used to performing the movements without overstressing them. As you improve, you can increase the total number of sets you complete. Experienced lifters often get better strength and hypertrophy (muscle growth) results by doing higher numbers of sets with fewer repetitions. That's why the ACSM guidelines for advanced weight trainers suggest doing 3-6 sets of up to 12 reps to maximise hypertrophy.

Tempo

The number of sets and reps you perform isn't the only variable that determines the training effect you'll get from your workouts. The speed at which you complete each phase of a rep also plays a part. Doing ten repetitions of a biceps curl, for example, as fast as possible won't have the same effect on your muscles

How reps affect your training

Rep Count:														
1	2	3	4	5	6	7	8	9	10	11	12	13	14	15+

Training effect:
Strength   **Hypertophy**   **Endurance**

■ Strength   ■ Hypertophy   ■ Endurance

as doing the move slowly.

To maximise strength and size gains, conditioning research suggests that your muscles should be under tension for between 40 to 70 seconds per set, provided you're not using extremely low repetition ranges. Lifting in this way will cause you to use anaerobic energy, which produces lactate and prompts the release of testosterone and growth hormones.

It's also important to use the right lifting speed within a rep. To make sure your muscles are under tension for long enough, take one second to lift the weight, pause then take two to three seconds to lower. The reason you should take longer to lower the weight is that size gains are best made during the eccentric (lowering) phase of the lift. Taking your time will also help you recruit stabilising muscles, which protect your joints and support your bigger muscles when you attempt heavy lifts. Another benefit is that slower lifting takes momentum out of the exercise.

Some exercises, however, such as the snatch, have to be performed at speed because they require explosive movements to lift a weight that's heavy enough for you to get a training benefit. As with sets and reps, it's also important to vary the tempo, so try to avoid using the same speed for every exercise and every workout.

Rest

The rest you take determines whether or not you're able to complete the next section of your workout. As a rule, sets with few reps will require the most rest. This is because they train the nervous system and fast-twitch muscle fibres, which fatigue easily and ke

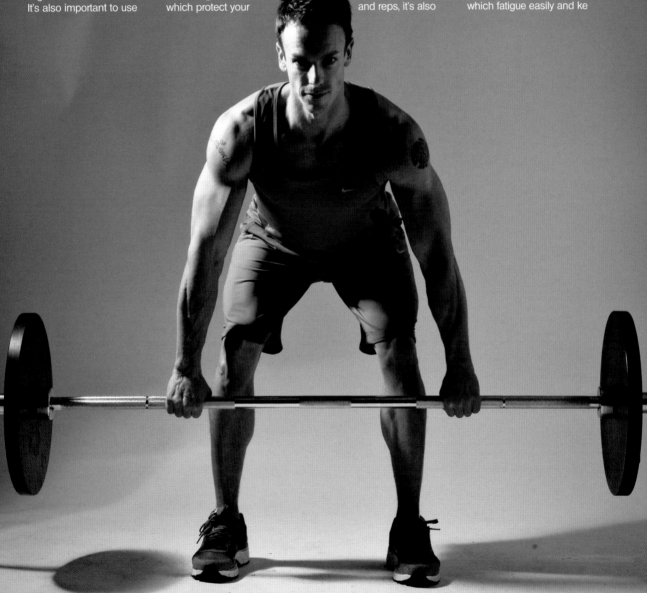

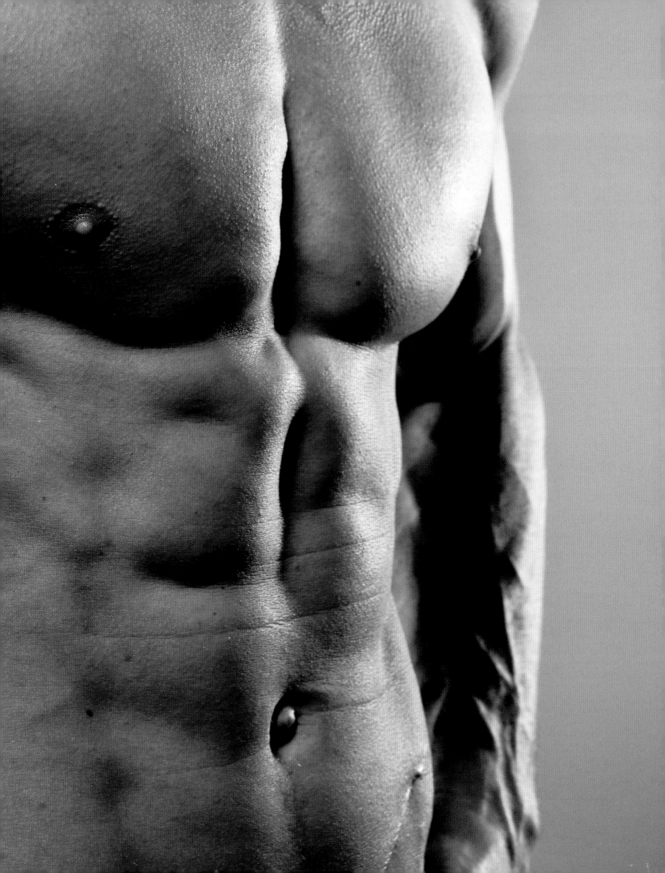

Training principles **I** Getting started

minutes when you perform very low reps of an explosive move with heavy weights. As you increase the number of reps you train your slow twitch muscle fibres, which are harder to fatigue.

Different exercises also require different rest times. Big compound moves such as squats and deadlifts require longer rests of about two minutes than single-joint isolation moves, which may only require 30 seconds rest between exercises.

Those new to weight training may need to take longer rests than more experienced lifters, who have a higher tolerance to the lactate produced during lifts. How much you weigh can also affect your rest times, with heavier lifters needing longer to recover between sets.

Essentially, your rest periods are effective when you can reach positive failure on the last rep of the set. This means that you are unable to lift the weight with perfect form but are able to lower it under control. If you don't reach that point by the end of your set, your rest may be too long.

It's also important to remember that rest is the same as any other training variable and that you should change the rest you take to stimulate your body into new muscle growth.

Selecting and ordering exercises

The exercises you should perform depend on what you want to achieve. The sample workouts in each of the kit chapters will give you an example of how to select exercises according to goals such as developing a particular body part, losing fat

or developing explosive power.

Structuring your workout properly is important because various exercises place different demands on your body. Some work multiple muscle groups, whereas some isolate small muscle groups. The speed, pattern of movement and body parts targeted should all influence how you order your exercises. The following guidelines will help you to structure your workouts to maximise muscle growth and strength gains and to minimise injury risk.

Do big explosive moves early in your workout

Explosive exercises such as the hang clean are very demanding so they need to be performed when you are relatively fresh. Do these moves earlier in your workout than simpler moves such as triceps extensions.

Do difficult moves first and easier moves last

Complete large muscle group moves, such as squats and deadlifts, at the beginning of your workout to make sure you keep perfect form and your core is strong enough to stabilise your body. Easier moves, such as biceps curls, should be done later in the workout.

Keep your workouts balanced

Unless you are specifically doing an unbalanced workout (made up, for example, exclusively of pushing movements), try to keep your workouts balanced. So, for every pushing exercise you do, you should do a pulling one.

Save core moves until last

If you do core moves early on

in your workout you'll fatigue the muscles. When you then come to do big dynamic lifts, such as lunges, that call on your core to stabilise your movement, they may not be able to provide adequate support, which can increase your injury risk.

Frequency

How many workouts you do per week is often influenced by work and family commitments. The good news, if you lead a busy life, is that you don't need to work out seven days a week to see great results. Doing from three to five workouts per week should be sufficient to achieve your workout goals.

Exactly how many sessions you do depends on a number of factors. One thing that should influence training frequency is what sort of workouts you're doing. A hard fully-body session may mean that you need to leave at least 48 hours between sessions in order for your muscles to recover and repair themselves to be stronger then before. If you're focusing on a particular body part each workout, you may be able to train the following day if you work on a different body part.

One common mistake is to think that the more workouts you do, the stronger and more muscular you'll

become. In fact it's while you're resting, rather than while you're working out, that your muscles get bigger and stronger. If you stress your muscles before they've had a chance to repair themselves this may cause what's known as overtraining, where you lose strength and muscle mass and feel lethargic.

Some muscle groups take longer to recover than others. Larger muscle groups, particularly those with a comparatively higher percentage of fast-twitch muscle fibres, such as the hamstrings, may take longer to recover than smaller muscle groups such as the calves.

Doing big compound lifts such as deadlifts also places more of a stress on your nervous system than smaller lifts, such as wrist curls, so you'll need longer to recover. You should also take longer to recover from intense sessions, where you do low reps of heavy weights, than you do from endurance and stability sessions, where you do high reps of light weights.

The good news is that you don't have to work out seven days a week to see great results

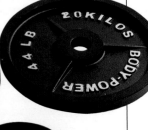

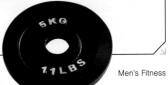

Getting started **I** Cardio

Improving your cardio fitness

Structure your cardio sessions to complement your weight training

You may think that adding long runs to your home workouts will complement your muscle building work. In fact, it can have the opposite effect. You see, while cardio training will improve your heart and lung function, and prepare your lower body for endurance events, it doesn't have a great effect on muscle size. Doing long, steady-state cardio sessions can even break down your muscle tissue, replacing your bulky fast-twitch fibres with slender slow-twitch ones that are better suited to pounding the pavements for mile after mile. Weight training is good for building muscles but it doesn't offer all the benefits you get from running, swimming or cycling. To make sure you get the best of both worlds, follow these rules:

1 Don't do weights and cardio back to back
If your main goal is to build muscle, keep weights sessions and cardio sessions separate. Doing cardio immediately before a weights session will leave you feeling tired and will lead to poor lifting performance. Doing cardio straight after a weights session can undo the muscle-building effects of a workout. The answer is to do them on separate days, which gives your muscles time to recover between sessions.

2 Keep cardio sessions short and intense
When you start a run (or any other type of cardio activity), your body uses energy from its own fat supplies and the food that you've eaten. After about 45 minutes of exercise it then switches to take energy from your muscles, and will eventually break down muscle tissue as you steadily plod away. The solution, unsurprisingly, is to keep your cardio sessions to under 45 minutes. To avoid losing out on the cardio benefits of a long run, make your sessions intense – and the best way to do this is by doing intervals. An interval session involves periods of intense activity followed by periods of lower intensity recovery. Try the interval session in the box below. As your fitness improves, you can increase the duration or intensity of intervals without lengthening the session.

3 Keep eating
The right nutrition is vital to achieving the body you want. If you're doing both weight training and cardio it becomes even more important because you need to fuel your exertions in the cardio sessions and still have enough calories to build the muscle you've trained so hard for. For more nutrition advice, go to page 176.

Sample interval run
Welcome to the pyramid interval

This session builds your bursts of speed up gradually and tapers off at the end as your energy levels are dwindling. Use a running watch to time your intervals. If you can't complete the session, do as much as you can and do more as you improve.

- **10** minutes easy jog
- **30** seconds fast, **60** seconds recovery
- **30** seconds fast, **60** seconds recovery
- **60** seconds fast, **60** seconds recovery
- **60** seconds fast, **60** seconds recovery
- **90** seconds fast, **60** seconds recovery
- **90** seconds fast, **60** seconds recovery
- **60** seconds fast, **60** seconds recovery
- **60** seconds fast, **60** seconds recovery
- **30** seconds fast, **60** seconds recovery
- **30** seconds fast, **60** seconds recovery
- **10** minutes easy jog

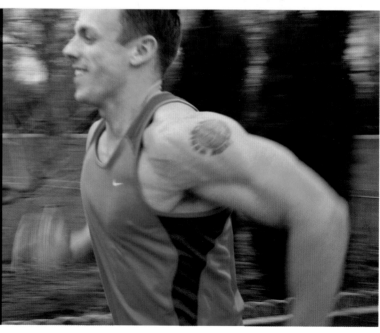

Know your muscles

The body has over 600 muscles. These are the key ones you'll target

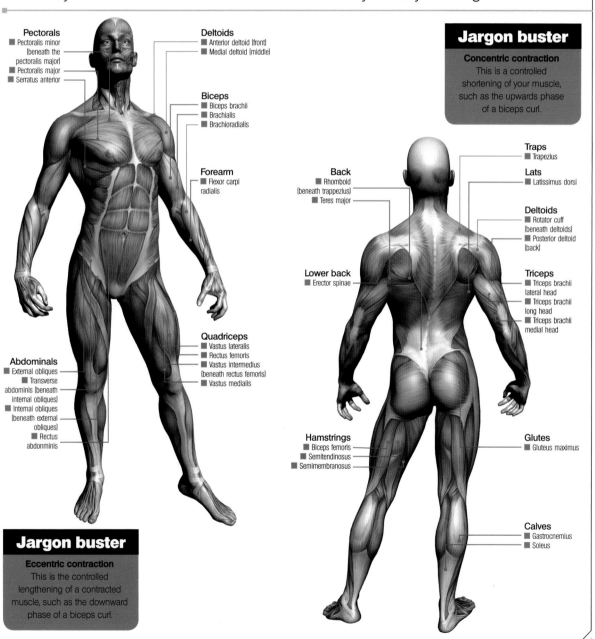

Pectorals
- Pectoralis minor (beneath the pectoralis major)
- Pectoralis major
- Serratus anterior

Deltoids
- Anterior deltoid (front)
- Medial deltoid (middle)

Biceps
- Biceps brachii
- Brachialis
- Brachioradialis

Forearm
- Flexor carpi radialis

Abdominals
- External obliques
- Transverse abdominis (beneath internal obliques)
- Internal obliques (beneath external obliques)
- Rectus abdonminis

Quadriceps
- Vastus lateralis
- Rectus femoris
- Vastus intermedius (beneath rectus femoris)
- Vastus medialis

Back
- Rhomboid (beneath trappezius)
- Teres major

Lower back
- Erector spinae

Hamstrings
- Biceps femoris
- Semitendinosus
- Semimembranosus

Traps
- Trapezius

Lats
- Latissimus dorsi

Deltoids
- Rotator cuff (beneath deltoids)
- Posterior deltoid (back)

Triceps
- Triceps brachii lateral head
- Triceps brachii long head
- Triceps brachii medial head

Glutes
- Gluteus maximus

Calves
- Gastrocnemius
- Soleus

Jargon buster

Concentric contraction
This is a controlled shortening of your muscle, such as the upwards phase of a biceps curl.

Jargon buster

Eccentric contraction
This is the controlled lengthening of a contracted muscle, such as the downward phase of a biceps curl.

Getting started | Warm-up

Pre-workout warm-up

Get your body ready for muscle growth and reduce your injury risk with this quick pre-workout warm-up

The warm-up is one of the most neglected aspects of a workout. It can seem like a boring waste of time but doing a proper warm-up will help you avoid injury and get the most out of the meat of your session.

The purpose of a warm-up is simple: to raise your core temperature and prepare your muscles for the work to come. Doing some light cardiovascular exercise, such as jogging on the spot, will make your heart beat faster, which pumps oxygen and nutrients to your muscles and elevates your body's temperature. Warm muscles are more elastic, which means you can work them through a fuller range of motion to get the best results from your exercises.

Once you've done that, do a few dynamic stretches (described opposite). These will target the muscles you'll use during the workout so they're primed for heavy lifting. Dynamic stretches involve moving continuously, placing the muscle under more tension with each repetition, which prepares your muscle joints and nerves for the actions they're about to perform. They differ from static stretches (see pages 22-23), which, according to the latest research, should not be done before a workout. A recent study found that pre-workout static stretches reduce the power available to a muscle during the workout, which has a negative effect on strength gains.

When you start your workout you should perform a 'warm-up set' of each exercise, where you do the move with a light weight. This will allow you to make sure your form is correct but does not count as one of the sets you plan to perform.

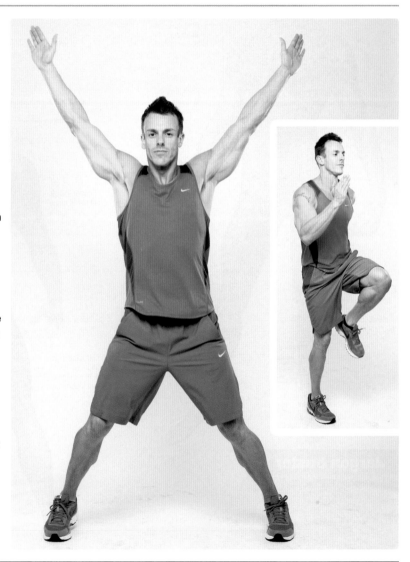

Warm-up I Getting started

Warm-up dynamic stretches

Do ten repetitions of each of the following exercises, alternating sides with each rep where appropriate. Start gently and aim to increase the range of motion with each rep

01

Lunge with
reverse flye

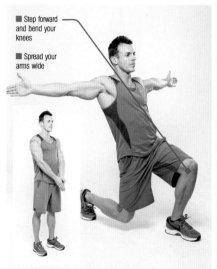

- Step forward and bend your knees
- Spread your arms wide

02

Lateral lunge
with twist

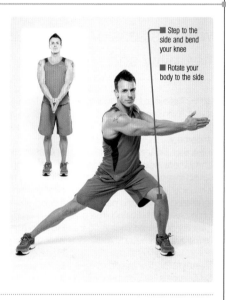

- Step to the side and bend your knee
- Rotate your body to the side

03

Alternating
split deadlift

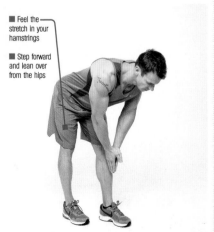

- Feel the stretch in your hamstrings
- Step forward and lean over from the hips

04

Squat to reach

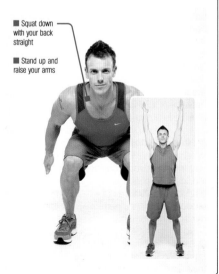

- Squat down with your back straight
- Stand up and raise your arms

Getting started I Stretching

Post-workout stretch

Do the following stretches after a weights session to increase your flexibility and reduce injury risk

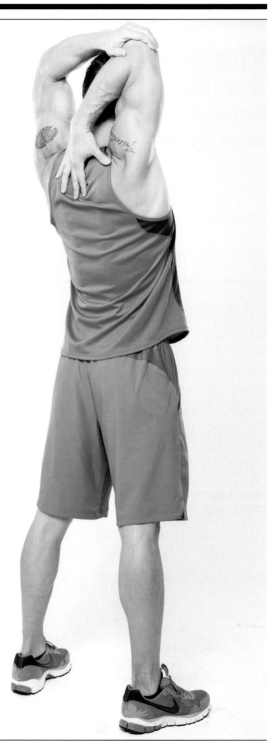

Post-workout stretching is an area of weight training that divides expert opinion. Some coaches think that it offers no benefits and others recommend static stretching, where you relax a muscle and hold it under tension for a specific period of time without moving. The majority advocate stretching at the end of a workout.

Benefits of stretching

Static stretches lengthen the muscle after it has contracted as a result of weight training and give you the following benefits:

■ Greater flexibility

Regular stretching will allow you to perform exercises across a wider range of movement, giving you greater muscle-building effect.

■ Fewer injuries

When you have less tension in your muscles you significantly reduce your chances of tearing muscle fibres or tendons when you perform dynamic movements.

■ Faster recovery

Stretching improves blood flow to your muscles and helps to flush out toxins, meaning you will be ready for your next workout sooner.

■ Better posture

Tense muscles can pull your shoulders, hips and spine out of alignment, which can cause back pain.

How to stretch

After you've finished your workout spend five minutes doing some gentle cardio, such as jogging on the spot, to bring your heart rate down. Then perform the stretches opposite, paying particular attention to the ones that target the muscles you worked during your session.

Get into the stretch position and allow your muscle to relax. As you place pressure on your muscle you should be able to feel it relaxing and lengthening.

You can slowly increase the pressure on the muscle throughout the duration of the stretch but you should never force it or 'bounce' because that can damage the muscle.

Hold each stretch for between 15 and 30 seconds but if you feel pain, stop immediately to avoid making a potential injury worse.

Stretching I Getting started

Calves

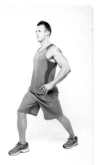

Take a step forward and press your back heel down to feel the stretch in your rear calf.

Hamstrings

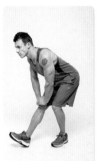

Keep your front leg straight and lean forward to feel the stretch in the hamstring of your front leg.

Quads

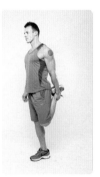

Hold your ankle and push your hips forward to feel the stretch in your thigh.

Hip flexors

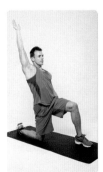

Step forward into a lunge so that your back knee is in contact with the ground. Keep your body upright and push your hips forward.

Adductors

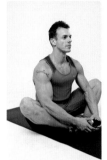

Touch your soles together and press gently on your knees with your elbows.

Glutes

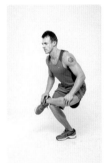

Stand on one leg and balance the bottom of your raised shin on your standing knee. Sink down until you feel the stretch in your glutes.

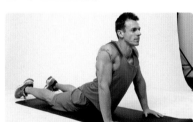

Abs

Lie on a mat with palms under your shoulders and your elbows tucked in. Then raise your shoulders while keeping your hips on the ground.

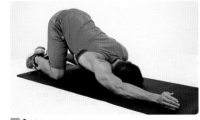

Lats

Kneel down and extend one arm out so it rests on the ground. Press down on your leading arm to feel the stretch down your side.

Lower back

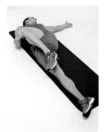

Keeping your shoulders flat on the floor, bend one knee at 90° and rotate your hips to send one leg over the other, pressing down to feel the stretch.

Chest

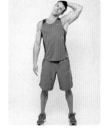

With your palms facing forwards, take your arms back to feel the stretch across your chest.

Traps

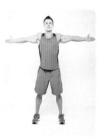

Pull gently on your head and pull your opposite shoulder down.

Triceps

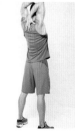

Bend one arm at the elbow and drop it down behind your back. With your other arm, push down gently on your elbow.

Biceps

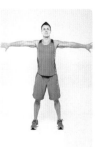

With your palms facing backwards, press your arms behind you to feel the stretch in your biceps.

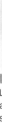
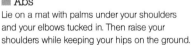

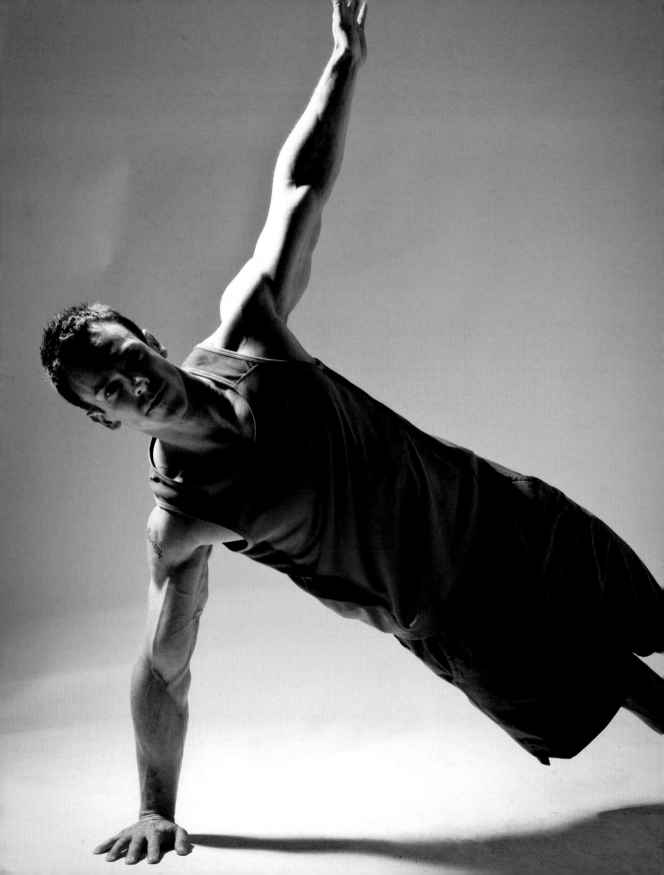

Bodyweight
introduction

Start building muscle right now just by using your bodyweight

If you've bought this book but haven't yet got round to buying any workout kit, don't worry. You can start building muscle straight away by doing bodyweight exercises.

For a muscle to grow in size and strength, it has to move against resistance (in this case, yourself), to create microscopic tears in the muscle fibres. These fibres will heal to be bigger and stronger than before. You still have to follow the training principles outlined in the previous chapter so you may need to adjust your tempo, for example, if you want to work in a muscle-building rep range. If you do that, you can start gaining muscle before you've bought any kit.

This chapter begins by demonstrating moves that will target different muscles. Once you know how to do the moves, we'll show you how to put them together to achieve your particular muscle building goals.

Bodyweight exercises such as one-leg squats are good at developing joint stability because you have to push a significant level of resistance while balancing on one leg. Controlling your own bodyweight will also give you practical strength because you're working with the load you carry around in everyday life.

There are lots of bodyweight moves you can do to target your core muscles, which you'll need to develop if you want to progress safely to doing big lifts such as a lunges with dumb-bells and even a barbell.

You can use bodyweight exercises to target any muscle group although, as you improve, you'll find it increasingly difficult to achieve the overload that will lead to muscle growth. When that happens, introducing some of the basic bits of kit outlined in later chapters will help you avoid getting stuck in a training rut. You should, however, still include bodyweight exercises in some of your workouts because you need to constantly refresh and tweak the way you work out to make sure your muscles are stimulated.

Bodyweight **Exercises**

01

Chair dip

Target: triceps
Develop your triceps with this compound bodyweight move, which will also improve shoulder joint stability.

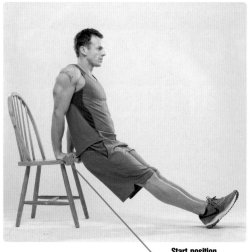

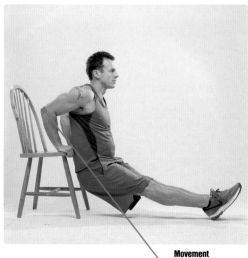

Start position
- Grip the edge of the chair with your hands
- Keep your feet together and legs straight and your back upright

Movement
- Lower your body straight down, keeping your elbows pointing back then press back up powerfully

02

Chair dip with leg lift

Target: triceps, core
Raising your leg introduces a rotational element to the exercise, which calls on your core to stabilise the movement.

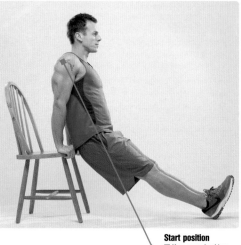

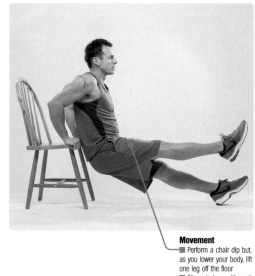

Start position
- Keep your shoulders back and your core braced

Movement
- Perform a chair dip but, as you lower your body, lift one leg off the floor
- Alternate legs with each repetition

Exercises | Bodyweight

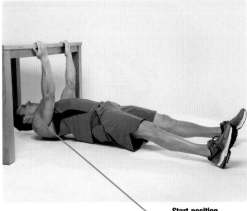

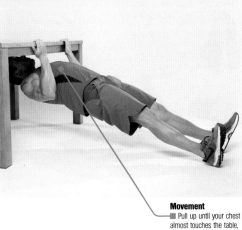

03

Table chin-up

Target: biceps, lats, forearms
Use a table as a prop to build your biceps.

Start position
- Lie under a solid table and grip the edges above your shoulders
- Keep your body in a straight line from head to heels

Movement
- Pull up until your chest almost touches the table, pause for a second while you squeeze your shoulder blades together then return slowly to the start

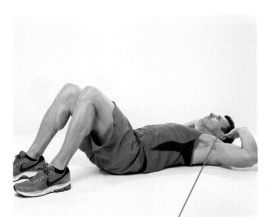

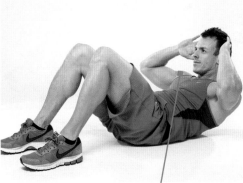

04

Crunch

Target: upper abdominals
Work your abs to build a solid six-pack with this classic mid-section move.

Start position
- Rest your fingers on your temples and don't pull your neck
- Hold your head off the floor
- Bend your knees at 90° and keep your feet flat on the floor

Movement

- Contract your abs to lift your shoulders off the floor
- Keep your lower back in contact with the floor and curl your chest towards your knees
- Pause at the top of the move to squeeze your abs and lower slowly to the start

Fit Tip

Don't do sit-ups

Using something to keep your feet in place works your hip flexor muscles. Crunches are much more effective at targeting your six-pack.

Bodyweight I **Exercises**

Reverse crunch

Target: lower abdominals

Hit your easily neglected lower abs with this simple move.

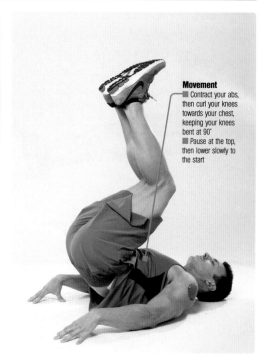

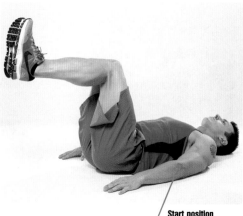

Movement
- Contract your abs, then curl your knees towards your chest, keeping your knees bent at 90˚
- Pause at the top, then lower slowly to the start

Start position
- Keep your head and shoulders on the floor and your arms by your sides
- Your thighs should be vertical and your knees should be bent at 90˚

Oblique crunch

Target: obliques

Work your side abs to for a fuller development of your abdominals.

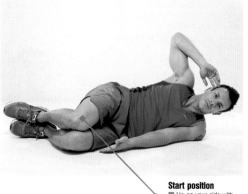

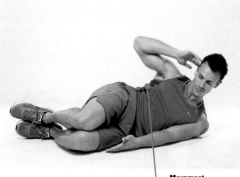

Start position
- Lie on your side with one arm in front of you, bending your knees for stability
- Touch your fingers to your temples on the side you're going to crunch

Movement
- Use your side abs to crunch up sideways, pause at the top of the move and lower slowly to the start

Exercises **|** Bodyweight

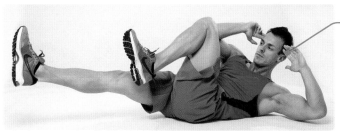

Start position
■ Start with your fingers by your temples and crunch up to bring your right elbow to your left knee while extending your right leg

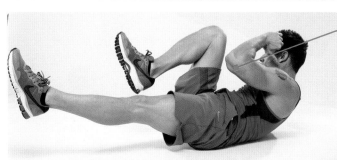

Movement
■ Twist your torso to the other side to bring your left elbow to you right knee while extending your left leg
■ Use your abs to control the move and try not to strain at the neck

07

Bicycles

Target:
abdominals
Use this dynamic move to hit your mid section from a range of angles.

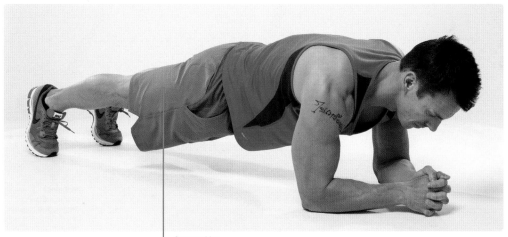

08

Plank

Target: core
Develop the muscles that support your spine with this classic static stability move.

Start position
■ Position yourself so that your feet are together and your body is straight from head to heels with your elbows underneath your shoulders and your head looking down
■ Hold the position as long as possible without letting your hips sag

Bodyweight **I** Exercises

09

Side plank

Target: core
Hold the plank in a different way to target your core muscles from a new angle.

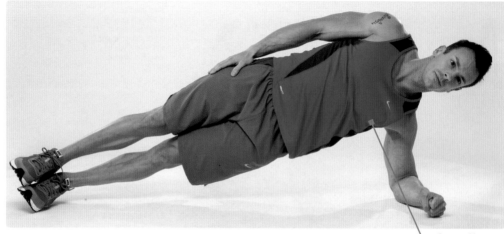

Start position
- Position yourself so that your elbow is directly underneath your shoulder and your body is in a straight line from head to heels
- Hold the position for as long as you can without letting your hips drop, then repeat it on the other side

10

Side plank star

Target: core
By raising your arm and leg your bring other muscles into the move and increase the challenge to your core.

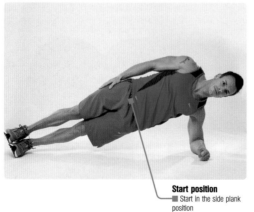

Start position
- Start in the side plank position

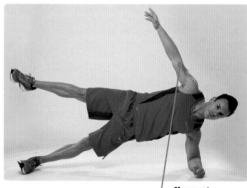

Movement
- Simultaneously raise your top arm and leg
- Hold that position for as long as possible and don't let your hips sag

Fit Tip

Do more than crunch

For an all-round abs routine include flexion exercises such as a crunch, two-point box, oblique crunches, woodchop and static holds such as the plank.

Exercises | Bodyweight

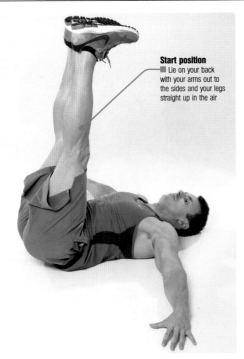

Start position
- Lie on your back with your arms out to the sides and your legs straight up in the air

Movement
- Twist over to one side, keeping your legs straight and your shoulders on the floor
- Don't let your feet touch the floor and alternate sides with each rep

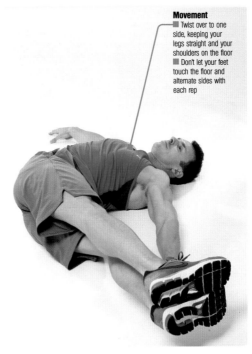

11

Lower-body Russian twist

Target: lower abdominals

By transferring the rotation to your lower abdominals you can do this move without any kit.

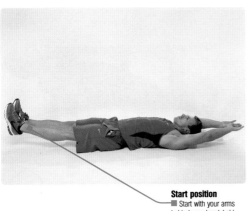

Start position
- Start with your arms behind your head, held off the floor, and your feet together, also off the floor

Movement
- Contract your abs to bring your arms and legs up to meet above your stomach, keeping your legs as straight as you can
- Squeeze your abs hard at the top of the move and lower to the start as slowly as you can

12

Jackknife

Target: upper and lower abdominals

This move requires a strong core to maintain perfect form and is great for developing a large part of your abs.

Bodyweight **I** Exercises

13

Squat thrusts

Target: core, quads

Get your heart rate up and work your core with this tiring move, which is also good for developing leg speed.

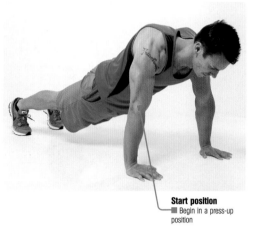

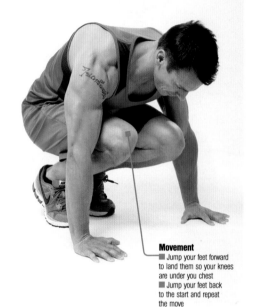

Start position
- Begin in a press-up position

Movement
- Jump your feet forward to land them so your knees are under you chest
- Jump your feet back to the start and repeat the move

14

Table pull-up

Target: mid-traps, lats, rhomboids

Use your bodyweight and a simple prop to build a muscular back.

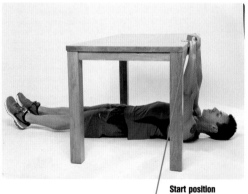

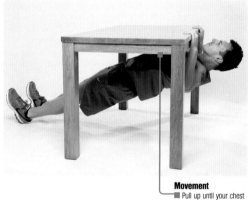

Start position
- Lie under a solid table and grip the edges above your shoulders so your fingers are pointing away from you

Movement
- Pull up until your chest touches the table, pause for a second while you squeeze your shoulder blades together, then return slowly to the start

Exercises | Bodyweight

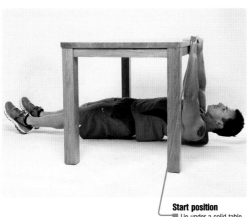

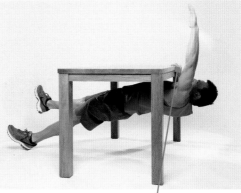

Table pull-up and reach

Target: mid-traps, lats, rhomboids, core

This move will build strength and take good core control to stabilise the movement.

Start position
- Lie under a solid table and grip the edges above your shoulders so your fingers are pointing away from you

Movement
- Pull up, then reach as high as you can with one hand
- Bring your hand back to the table and lower back down
- Alternate hands with each rep

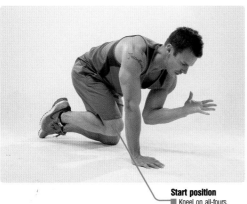

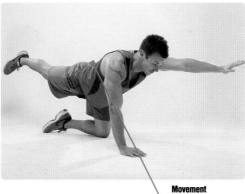

16

Two-point box

Target: lower back

This moves is excellent for strengthening the muscles that support your spine, which reduces your chances of injury during big lifts.

Start position
- Kneel on all-fours, then bring your elbow to meet your opposite knee beneath your stomach
- Keep looking down and stretch your arm and leg out straight

Movement
- Your body should form a straight line from foot to fingertips – don't let your hips rotate
- Hold that position for a count of two, return to the start and repeat on the opposite side

Bodyweight **I** Exercises

17

Dorsal raise with shoulder rotation

**Target:
lower back**

This move protects your lower back from injury and the twist at the top of the move intensifies the muscle contraction.

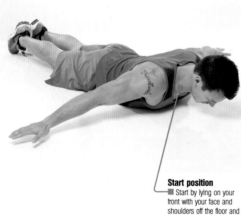

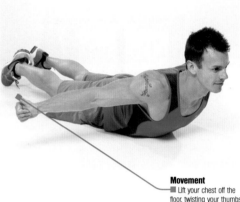

Start position
- Start by lying on your front with your face and shoulders off the floor and your arms out to the sides, palms facing down

Movement
- Lift your chest off the floor, twisting your thumbs back so they point towards the ceiling
- Squeeze your shoulder blades together at the top of the move

18

Press-up

Target: chest, triceps

Do this classic move to build your chest and arms.

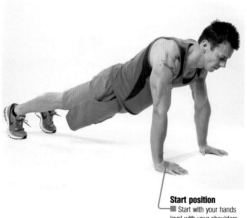

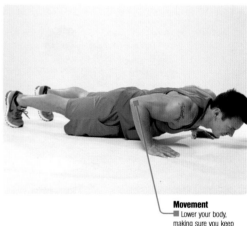

Start position
- Start with your hands level with your shoulders, just wider than shoulder-width apart
- Keep your body in a straight line from head to heels throughout the move

Movement
- Lower your body, making sure you keep your elbows pointing back rather than to the sides

Exercises I Bodyweight

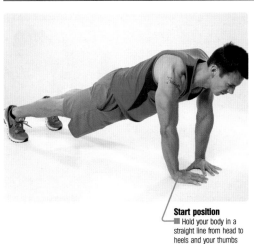

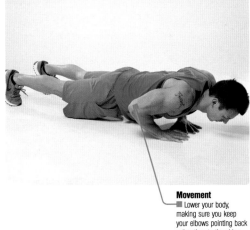

Start position
■ Hold your body in a straight line from head to heels and your thumbs and index fingers together to form a diamond shape

Movement
■ Lower your body, making sure you keep your elbows pointing back rather than to the sides

19

Diamond press-up

Target: triceps, chest

Placing your thumb and index fingers together shifts the emphasis on to your triceps.

A

Start position
■ Begin in the press-up position

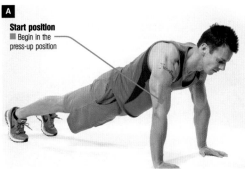

B

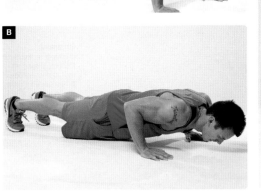

C

Movement
■ Lower down, keeping your elbows tucked in to your body (B)
■ Push up powerfully and twist your body, rolling on to the sides of your feet and keeping your body in a straight line
■ Raise one arm overhead with your arm straight then return to the start and perform the move on the opposite side

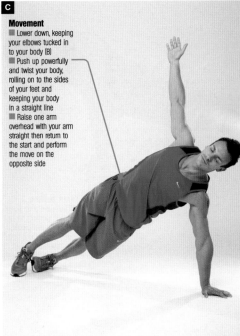

20

T press-up

Target: chest, core

Turn the press-up into an explosive move that works your body in more than one plane of motion.

Bodyweight I **Exercises**

21

Jump press-up

Target: chest, triceps
Develop your fast-twitch muscle fibres by pushing up explosively so both palms leave the floor.

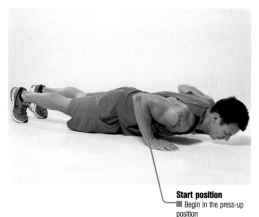

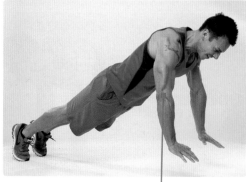

Start position
- Begin in the press-up position

Movement
- Lower down, keeping your elbows tucked in to your body
- Push up explosively so your hands leave the floor, land and go straight into the next jump press-up

22

Press-up with knee lift

Target: chest, triceps, core
Adding a knee lift to the press-up challenges your core because it's forced to stabilise your body in an awkward position.

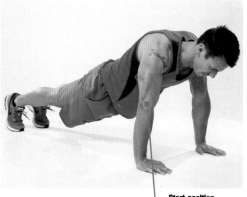

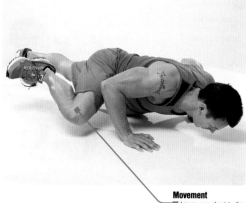

Start position
- Get into a press-up position with your hands beneath your shoulders and your body in a straight line from head to heels

Movement
- Lower your chest to the floor while bringing one knee up to your elbow
- Take care not to rotate your body as you lift your knee and alternate sides with each press-up

Exercises **I** Bodyweight

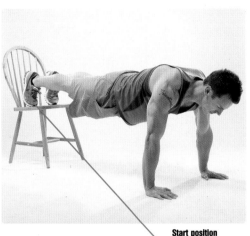

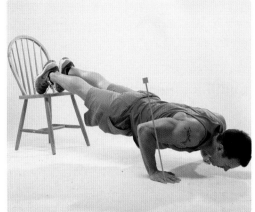

23

Decline press-up

Target: upper chest, triceps, shoulders
By raising your feet you place more of an emphasis on your upper chest.

Start position
- Get into a press-up position with your feet on a chair or box, your hands beneath your shoulders and your body in a straight line from head to heels

Movement
- Lower your upper body, keeping your elbows pointing back, not out, until your nose almost touches the floor then push back up

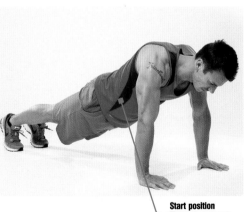

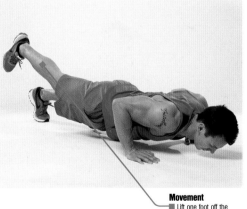

24

One-leg press-up

Target: chest, triceps, core
Keeping one leg raised while you perform the move will challenge your core because you're trying to keep stable while balancing on one leg.

Start position
- Get into a press up position with your hands beneath your shoulders and your body in a straight line from head to heels

Movement
- Lift one foot off the floor and lower your chest to the floor, keeping your elbows pointing back rather than out
- Complete your reps for that set and swap legs each set

Bodyweight I Exercises

25

Squat

Target: quads, glutes, hamstrings
This classic lower body move will build muscle and stabilise your ankle, knee and hip joints.

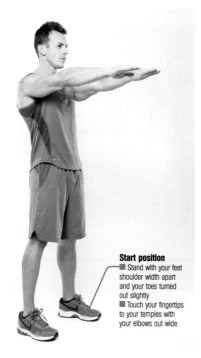

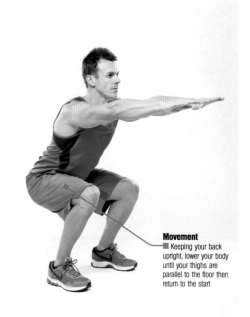

Start position
- Stand with your feet shoulder width apart and your toes turned out slightly
- Touch your fingertips to your temples with your elbows out wide

Movement
- Keeping your back upright, lower your body until your thighs are parallel to the floor then return to the start

26

One-leg squat

Target: quads, glutes, hamstrings
Doing the move on one leg ensures you get balanced muscle development as well as improving your stability, coordination and leg-pushing power.

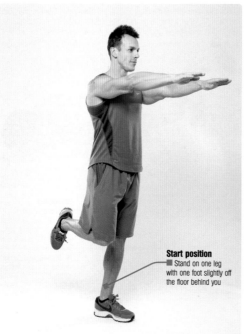

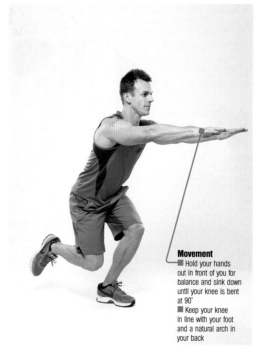

Start position
- Stand on one leg with one foot slightly off the floor behind you

Movement
- Hold your hands out in front of you for balance and sink down until your knee is bent at 90˚
- Keep your knee in line with your foot and a natural arch in your back

Exercises | Bodyweight

Start position
- Lower into a squat then push off explosively to jump off the ground

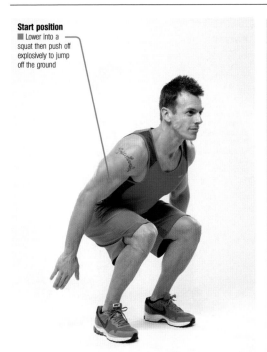

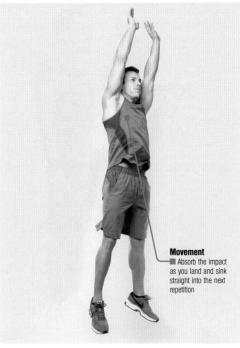

Squat jump

Target: quads, glutes, hamstrings
This move develops explosive power, which is useful for activities such as sprinting.

Movement
- Absorb the impact as you land and sink straight into the next repetition

Start position
- Position yourself so your shoulders and hips are pressed against the wall and your knees are bent at 90 degrees
- Hold the position for as long as you can without breaking good form

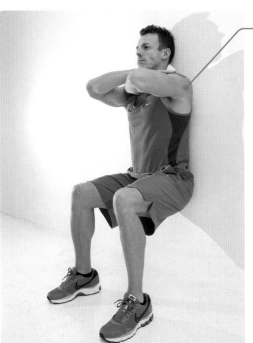

Wall squat

Target: quads, glutes, hamstrings
Holding this isometric position will flood your muscles with lactic acid so do it at the end of a workout to completely fatigue your legs.

Fit Tip

Wiggle when you squat

For squats and lunges, wiggle your toes at the base of the move. If you can't, it means your weight is too far forwards. Push up through your heels, not toes.

Bodyweight I Exercises

29

Lunge

Target: quads, hamstrings
This dynamic move tests your coordination and builds lower-body strength.

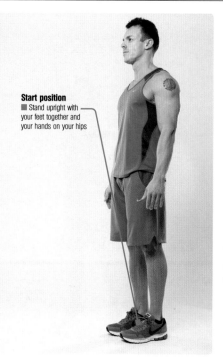

Start position
■ Stand upright with your feet together and your hands on your hips

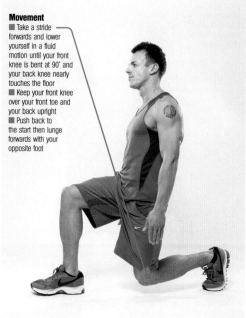

Movement
■ Take a stride forwards and lower yourself in a fluid motion until your front knee is bent at 90° and your back knee nearly touches the floor
■ Keep your front knee over your front toe and your back upright
■ Push back to the start then lunge forwards with your opposite foot

30

Lunge jump

Target: quads, hamstrings
Adding a jump to the move develops your explosive power while testing your balance and coordination.

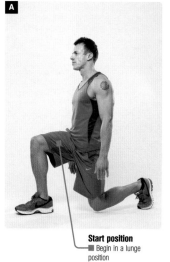

A

Start position
■ Begin in a lunge position

B

C

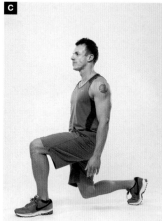

Movement
■ Jump up, swapping your leg positions in mid air
■ Land in the lunge position, absorbing the impact before going straight into the next lunge jump

Exercises | Bodyweight

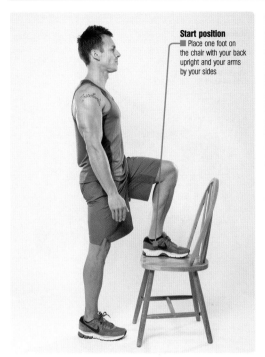

Start position
■ Place one foot on the chair with your back upright and your arms by your sides

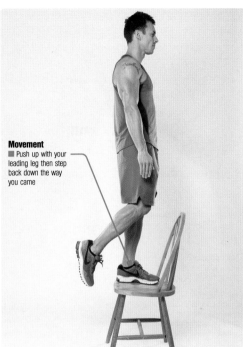

Movement
■ Push up with your leading leg then step back down the way you came

 31

Chair step-up

Target: glutes, quads
This exercise builds practical strength because it's similar to the movement you make when climbing stairs.

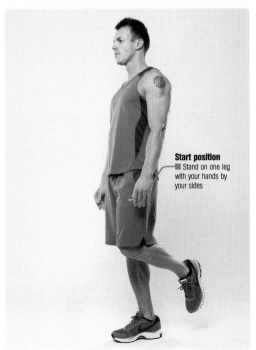

Start position
■ Stand on one leg with your hands by your sides

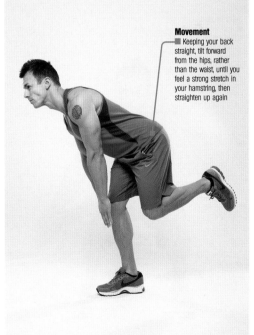

Movement
■ Keeping your back straight, tilt forward from the hips, rather than the waist, until you feel a strong stretch in your hamstring, then straighten up again

32

One-leg deadlift

Target: hamstrings
Strengthen the backs of your legs with this move that also improves your balance.

Bodyweight **I** Exercises

33

Inverted shoulder press

Target: shoulders
It's difficult to target your shoulders using bodyweight alone but this move will get them working.

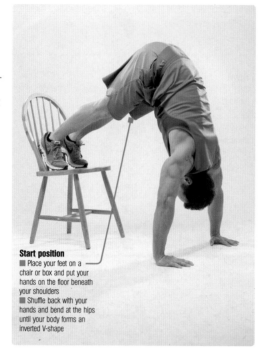

Start position
■ Place your feet on a chair or box and put your hands on the floor beneath your shoulders
■ Shuffle back with your hands and bend at the hips until your body forms an inverted V-shape

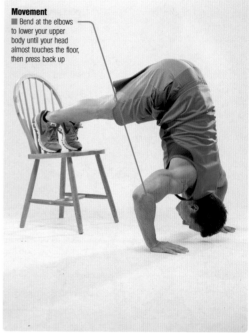

Movement
■ Bend at the elbows to lower your upper body until your head almost touches the floor, then press back up

34

Woodchop

Target: core, lower back, quads, shoulders
Develop your ability to transfer force from the lower to the upper half of your body with this sporty move.

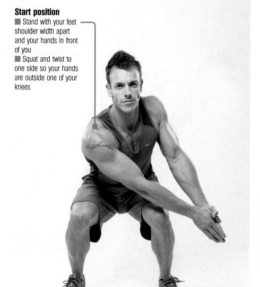

Start position
■ Stand with your feet shoulder width apart and your hands in front of you
■ Squat and twist to one side so your hands are outside one of your knees

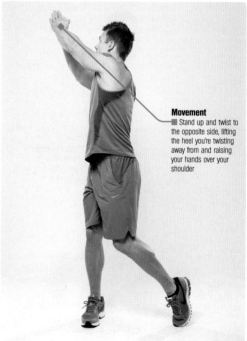

Movement
■ Stand up and twist to the opposite side, lifting the heel you're twisting away from and raising your hands over your shoulder

Workouts I Bodyweight

Full-body workout

The best thing about full-body workouts is that they allow you to work a large number of muscle fibres in a short space of time. The result is that your body releases a flood of growth hormones that will make your muscles get bigger and stronger. They're great if you're new to training because they get your muscles used to weight training without putting them under too much stress.

The downside of this workout is that it's hard to fully exhaust your muscle fibres.

Designing your workout
The key to a sound full-body workout is balance. That means making sure you have a pushing motion for every pulling motion you do and that you spend a roughly equal amount of time on your upper and lower body.

Opt for compound exercises (multi-joint moves that work several muscle groups at once), as these will give you maximum muscle-building benefits.

Leave abs specific exercises, such as the crunch, to the end of your workout because you don't want to exhaust your core muscles before they're called upon to stabilise your spine in more demanding moves such as a table pull-up.

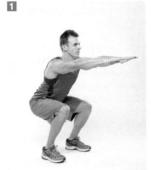
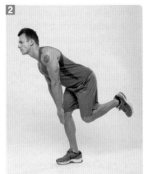
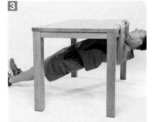
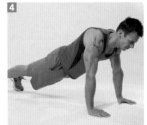
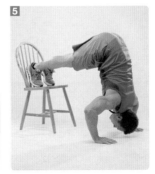
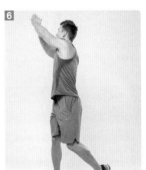
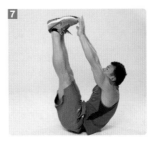

Full-body sample workout

1 Squat I **Sets: 3 Reps:** 10-12 **Page:** 38

2 One-leg deadlift I **Sets: 2 Reps:** 10 each side **Page:** 41

3 Table pull-up I **Sets: 3 Reps:** 10-12 **Page:** 32

4 Press-up I **Sets: 3 Reps:** 10-12 **Page:** 34

5 Inverted shoulder press I **Sets: 3 Reps:** 10-12 **Page:** 42

6 Woodchop I **Sets: 2 reps** 10 each side **Page:** 42

7 Jackknife I **Sets: 3 Reps:** 10-12 **Page:** 31

Bodyweight **I** Workouts

Circuit training

This is a great option if you're short on time or if your main goal is fat loss. By doing different exercises back to back with no rest in between you keep your effort level high and force your heart to pump blood to different parts of your body, giving you both a cardiovascular and a muscle building benefit. Circuits aren't the best way to build muscle but they will help you to look lean and defined.

Designing your workout

Circuits require you to move swiftly from one exercise to the next, which is easier with no kit. Aim to target as many different muscle groups as possible and alternate between upper and lower body moves to make your heart work harder without experiencing excessive muscle fatigue. Include a good mix of pushing, pulling, lunging, bending and rotational moves, to give your workout balance. You should also try to complete the reps quickly but without compromising good form. Once you have completed the circuit, rest for three minutes then do it all again. The fitter you become, the more circuits you'll be able to complete.

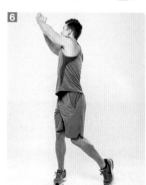

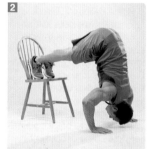

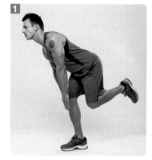

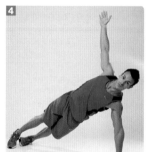

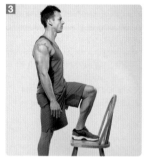

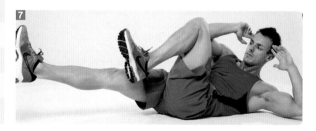

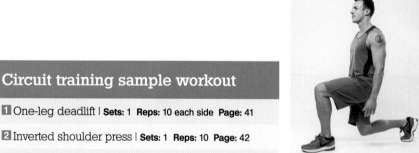

Circuit training sample workout

1 One-leg deadlift | **Sets: 1 Reps:** 10 each side **Page:** 41

2 Inverted shoulder press | **Sets: 1 Reps:** 10 **Page:** 42

3 Chair step-up
Sets: 1 Reps: 10 each side **Page:** 41

4 T-press-up | **Sets: 1 Reps:** 10 each side **Page:** 35

5 Lunge | **Sets: 1 Reps:** 10 each side **Page:** 40

6 Woodchop | **Sets: 1 Reps:** 10 each side **Page:** 42

7 Bicycles | **Sets: 1 Reps:** 0 each side **Page:** 29

Workouts | Bodyweight

Core stability workout

The term 'core stability' has become increasingly popular in recent years as strength coaches acknowledge the important role that the core muscles play in virtually every area of physical performance.

Your core muscles are the ones around your midriff, including your abs and lower back, and their function is to provide a link between your upper and lower body. They're particularly important during whole-body moves, which need a strong core to transfer power between the upper and lower halves of your body. They're also called upon to stabilise your spine during sporty movements such as running or kicking a football.

A weak core can cause lower back pain and poor posture. You may also find that you are ineffective at transferring power so the work you do on other muscle groups may be lost if your core lets you down.

Designing your workout

The mistake most men make when training their core and abdominal muscles is focusing too heavily on the upper abs by doing endless crunches. Instead, you need to place equal emphasis on training the muscles at the side and back of your midriff.

Target your core muscles from different angles, including rotational movements, for a thorough workout. Because this workout focuses on stability, you should complete a relatively high number of reps per set.

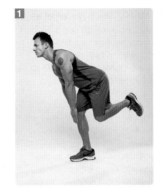

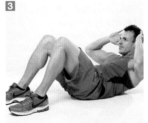

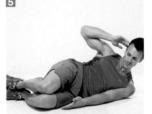

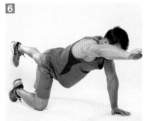

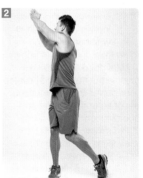

Core stability sample workout

1 One-leg deadlift | **Sets:** 2 **Reps:** 10-12 each side **Page:** 41

2 Woodchop | **Sets:** 2 **Reps:** 10-12 each side **Page:** 42

3 Crunch | **Sets:** 2 **Reps:** 15 **Page:** 27

4 Dorsal raise | **Sets:** 2 **Reps:** 15 **Page:** 34

5 Oblique crunch | **Sets:** 2 **Reps:** 15 each side **Page:** 28

6 Two-point box | **Sets:** 2 **Reps:** 15 each side **Page:** 33

7 Lower body Russian twist
Sets: 2 **Reps:** 15 each side **Page:** 31

Bodyweight I Workouts

Explosive power workout

Explosive workouts, also known as plyometric workouts, give you more than one type of benefit. They're good for building muscle but they'll also develop your power (the combination of speed and strength) and coordination.

Put simply, a plyometric exercise is one that involves extending a muscle across its full range of motion before explosively contracting it. This dynamic movement targets your fast-twitch muscle fibres, exhausting them quicker than a conventional workout but without having to add extra weight. The intensity will also raise your heart rate, burning extra calories and releasing muscle-building hormones.

These types of workouts are popular with sportsmen because they can be used to develop fast, powerful movements and improve skills, such as your vertical leap.

Designing your workout

For each target body part, start by doing an activation move to warm-up and stabilise your muscles. Then do the plyometric exercise before performing a single-joint move to exhaust the muscles.

The emphasis of these sessions is on speed and power, rather than developing endurance. This means it is essential for you to rest for at least one minute between sets and at least two minutes between exercises.

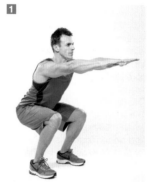

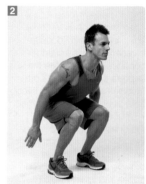

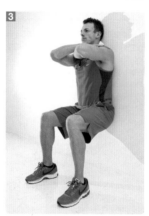

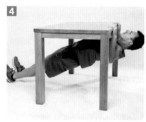

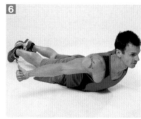

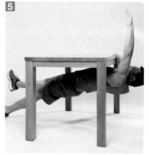

Explosive power sample workout:
legs and back

1 Squat I **Sets: 3 Reps: 12 Page: 38**

2 Squat jump I **Sets: 3 Reps: 10 Page: 39**

3 Static wall squat
Sets: 1 Time: hold as long as possible **Page: 39**

4 Table pull-up I **Sets: 3 Reps: 8 Page: 32**

5 Table pull up and reach
Sets: 2 Reps: 6 each side **Page: 33**

6 Dorsal raise I **Sets: 3 Reps: 10 Page: 34**

Workouts **|** Bodyweight

Superset workout

A superset is two exercises performed back to back with no rest in between. Once you have finished both exercises, you rest before performing the superset again, just as you would do with a regular set. The reason for doing supersets is that they are time efficient because you're reducing the amount of rest you take during a workout.

You can pair any two exercises to form a superset but the most popular option is to create 'antagonistic supersets', where the two moves work opposing body parts. An example would be to perform a press-up (which works your chest) then go straight into a table pull-up (which works your back). The advantage of antagonistic supersets is that they give one body part a chance to rest

while the opposing muscle group is working and they give you balanced muscle development. Other common forms include non-competing supersets, which target unrelated muscle groups, such as pairing a lower-body move with an upper-body one, and post-exhaustion supersets, where you do a multi-joint move followed by a single-joint move targeting the same body part.

Designing your workout
If you're going to do antagonistic supersets, for each exercise, find one that works its polar opposite, so if you do one exercise that targets your quads do another that targets your hamstrings. Biceps exercises should be paired with triceps moves, and so on. After each superset, rest for two minutes and repeat.

1 Superset A

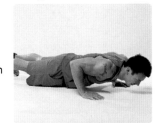

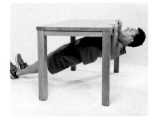

2 Superset B

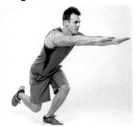

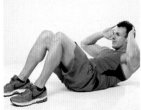

3 Superset C

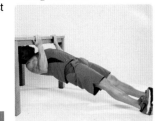

4 Superset D

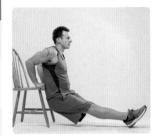

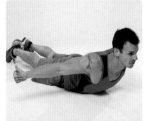

Superset sample workout

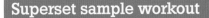

1 Superset A
Press-up I Table pull-up I **Sets:** 3 **Reps:** 10-12 **Page:** 34/32

2 Superset B
One-leg squat I One-leg deadlift
Sets: 2 each side **Reps:** 10-12 **Page:** 38/41

3 Superset C Table chin-up I Chair dip
Sets: 3 **Reps:** 10-12 **Page:** 27/26

4 Superset D Crunch I Dorsal raise
Sets: 3 **Reps:** 10-12 **Page:** 27/34

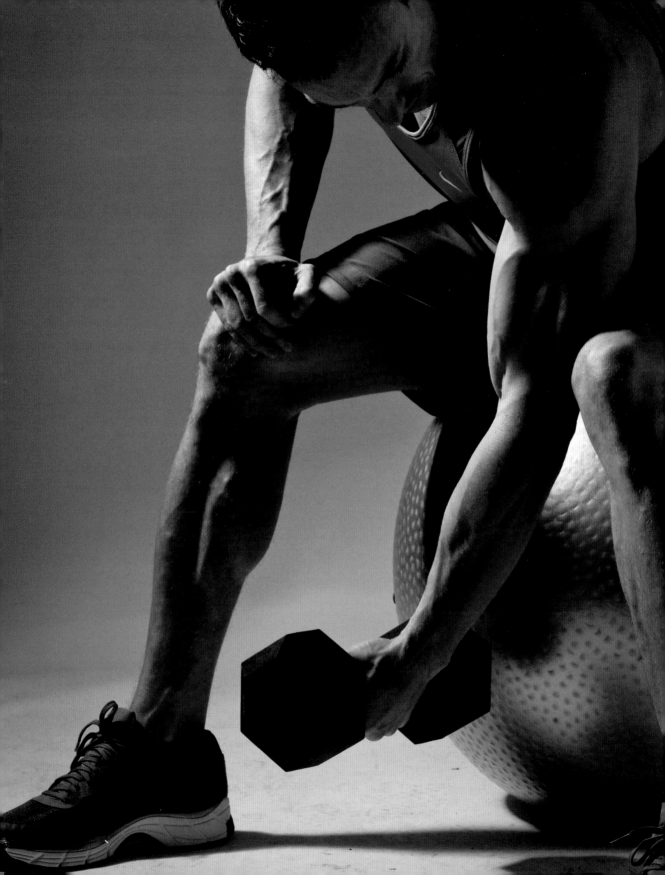

Dumb-bells & gym ball introduction

A set of dumb-bells and a gym ball can give you serious muscle gains

The foundation of any home gym set-up should be a set of dumb-bells and a gym ball. The reason they're so useful is that they are so versatile. You can target any body part in a variety of ways, increasing your chances of losing fat and gaining muscle.

This chapter will give you a wide variety of exercises for each major body part. You can then begin to explore a range of workout techniques that will make sure you keep challenging your body and help you get bigger and stronger.

Dumb-bells allow you to easily fatigue your muscles within your desired rep range, helping you to build new muscle. The fact that you hold one in each hand gives you balanced muscle growth and develops your stabilising muscles because you're forced to control their movement.

A gym ball is excellent at increasing the instability of an exercise, which will improve your core strength. The greater the instability, the harder the exercise. For that reason, a gym ball is a great tool to use in conjunction with a set of dumb-bells because you'll struggle to complete your sets of unstable exercises, even if your heaviest dumb-bell is 10kg.

Of course, there are some things that you can't do with dumb-bells and gym ball. If you want to do heavy compound lifts, which will burn lots of calories and flood your body with muscle growth hormones, you'll need to invest in a barbell and bench. But before you do that you need to build a solid base of fitness. And even once you introduce a bar and bench into your routine, you should still do dumb-bell and gym ball moves to get an all-round training effect.

Dumb-bells & gym ball I Buyer's guide

Dumb-bells and gym ball gear guide

A gym ball and a set of dumb-bells are the cornerstone of a home gym. Here's what they do and how to buy them

Gym ball

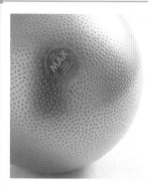

What it does

Gym balls, also known as stability balls or Swiss balls, promote increased joint and core stability by forcing the body to stabilise itself on an unstable surface. Stability balls are relatively cheap and portable so they're perfect for home training.

What to look for

Durability: Check that the ball is durable. The cheaper the ball, the more likely it is that you'll need to replace it after a few months, so buy one that's 'anti-burst'. You need to make sure it can support your bodyweight and additional weight such as a pair of dumb-bells.

Size: Gym balls come in different sizes. You want to be able to sit on top of the ball with your knees bent at about 90° and your feet flat on the floor, so taller people will need a larger size than shorter people. Use the following guide to find the right size:

User height	Ball size
1.50-1.64m	55cm
1.65-1.81m	65cm
1.82-2.00m	75cm

Dumb-bells

Dumb-bells allow you to perform an enormous number of resistance exercises. They're incredibly versatile and can be used to exhaust, and therefore develop, the strength and size of any muscle. Because you hold a dumb-bell in one hand it creates instability, which forces the body to control itself and encourages balanced muscle development. There are three main types of dumb-bell: fixed, plate-loaded and adjustable.

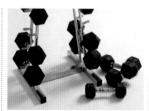

Fixed dumb-bells
As the name implies, the weight can't be altered. The advantage is that it's quick and easy to use your desired weight but the downside is that they're expensive and take up a lot of space. If you do invest in a set of fixed dumb-bells, try to get ones with hexagonal ends because they can be used on the floor for exercises such as T press-ups without rolling around.

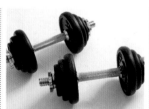

Plate-loaded dumb-bells
These are the low-cost option, so they're appealing if you're on a tight budget. They have two collars, which secure plates to either end of the dumb-bell bar. When they're loaded they work your body in exactly the same way as fixed and adjustable dumb-bells. The difference is that it can be time-consuming to keep altering the weights between exercises.

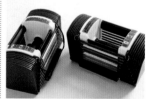

Adjustable dumb-bells
This type of dumb-bell lets you change the weight you lift without having to mess around with weight plates. The most sophisticated versions allow you to position a dial next to the value of the weight you want to lift. They are more expensive than plate-loaded dumb-bells but they're more convenient and they do allow you to stick rigidly to rest periods.

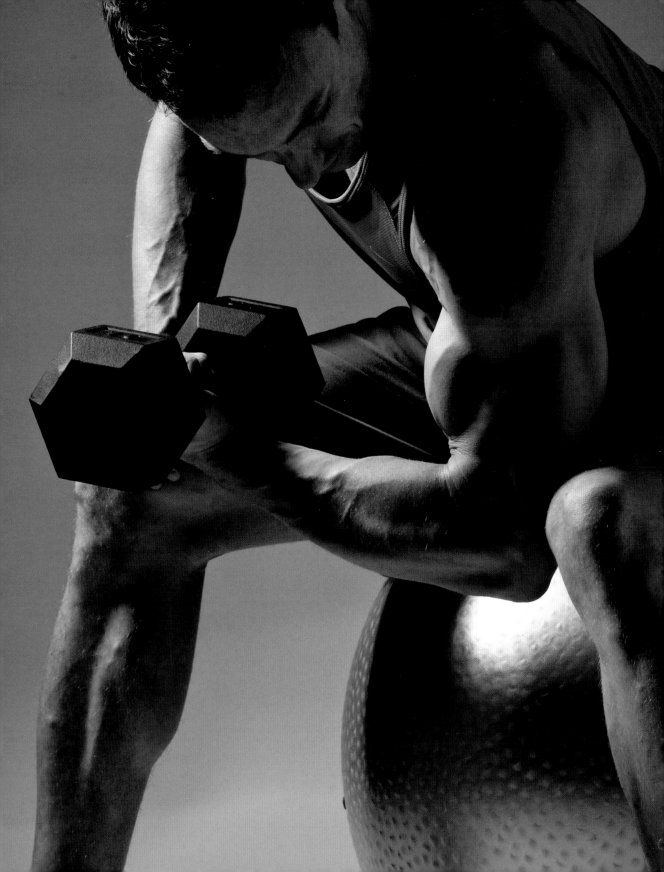

Dumb-bells & gym ball I **Exercises**

01

Dumb-bell curl

Target: biceps
Using dumb-bells will work your biceps evenly, giving you balanced muscle growth.

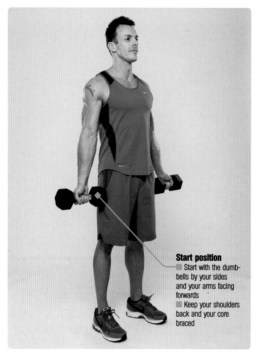

Start position
- Start with the dumb-bells by your sides and your arms facing forwards
- Keep your shoulders back and your core braced

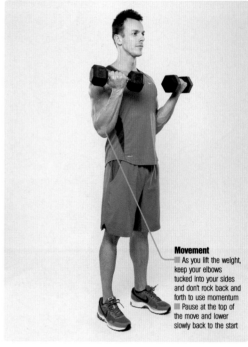

Movement
- As you lift the weight, keep your elbows tucked into your sides and don't rock back and forth to use momentum
- Pause at the top of the move and lower slowly back to the start

02

Gym ball dumb-bell curl

Target: biceps
Introducing a gym ball forces you to engage your core muscles to stabilse your body, which promotes good posture when performing the move without a ball.

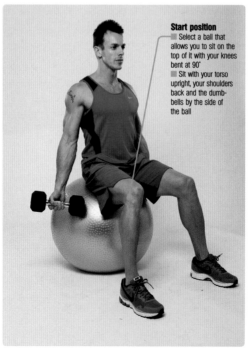

Start position
- Select a ball that allows you to sit on the top of it with your knees bent at 90°
- Sit with your torso upright, your shoulders back and the dumb-bells by the side of the ball

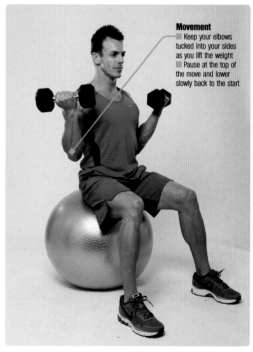

Movement
- Keep your elbows tucked into your sides as you lift the weight
- Pause at the top of the move and lower slowly back to the start

Exercises | Dumb-bells & gym ball

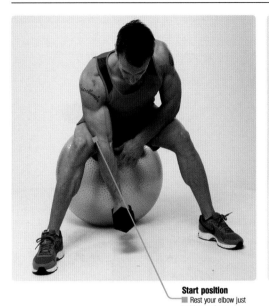

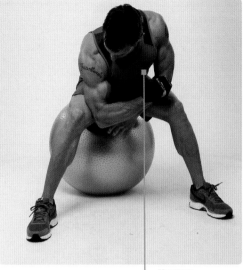

03

Concentration curl

Target: biceps
By locking your elbow in place you remove any upper-arm swing and focus the stress on your biceps.

Start position
- Rest your elbow just inside your knee

Movement
- Keep your upper body still and curl the dumb-bell up to your chest

Fit Tip

Stretch your triceps to build your biceps

To get the most out of your biceps moves, do a triceps stretch before each set of bicep curls to temporarily weaken the triceps. Provided you follow good form on the bicep curls, you should be able to get bigger arms, faster.

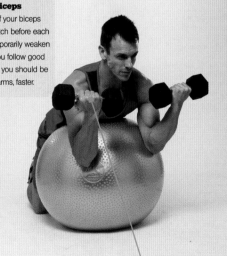

04

Gym ball dumb-bell preacher curl

Target: biceps
As well as hitting your biceps, this is a great move for developing coordination of your shoulders, hips and core in the frontal plane of motion. Use a lighter weight to make sure you perform the move correctly.

Start position
- Rest your upper arms on the ball and keep a slight bend in your elbows
- Turn your wrists inwards slightly to take some of the stress off that joint

Movement
- Keep your upper body still and curl the weights up towards your shoulders before lowering slowly to the start

Dumb-bells & gym ball **|** Exercises

Hammer curl

Target: biceps
Curling the weight with a neutral grip takes some of the emphasis off your biceps and places more stress on your forearms.

Start position
■ Stand with your back straight, your shoulders back and your core braced
■ Grip the dumb-bells with palms facing inwards and tuck your elbows into your sides

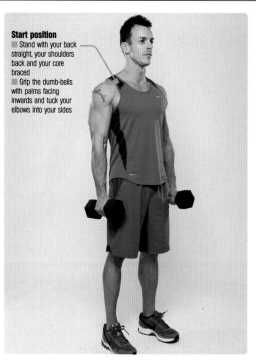

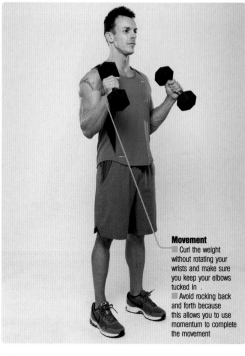

Movement
■ Curl the weight without rotating your wrists and make sure you keep your elbows tucked in .
■ Avoid rocking back and forth because this allows you to use momentum to complete the movement

Hammer curl with twist

Target: biceps
Performing the move one arm at a time encourages you to stay upright and take momentum out of the move. By rotating your wrists at the top of the move, you target your biceps from two angles.

Start position
■ Stand with your back straight, your shoulders back and your core braced
■ Grip the dumb-bells with palms facing inwards and tuck your elbows into your sides

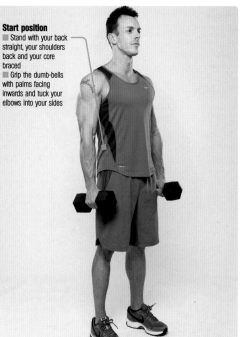

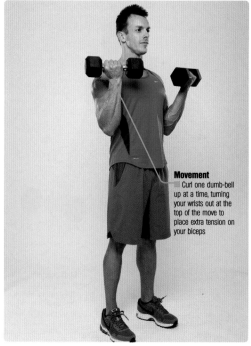

Movement
■ Curl one dumb-bell up at a time, turning your wrists out at the top of the move to place extra tension on your biceps

Exercises I Dumb-bells & gym ball

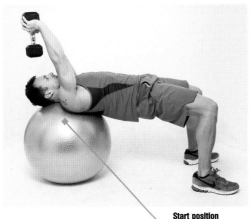

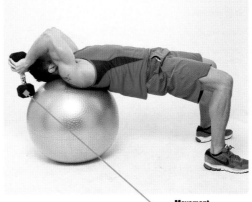

07

Gym ball lying triceps extension

Target: triceps, core
Doing a triceps extension on a gym ball calls on your core muscles to stabilise the movement.

Start position
■ Start with your upper back and shoulders in contact with the ball and hold a single dumb-bell above your face with both hands

Movement
■ Lower the weight behind your head, pivoting at the elbows to keep your upper arms still
■ Keep your body horizontal and your knees bent at 90˚

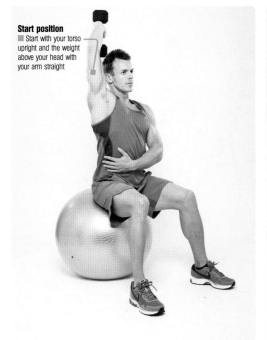

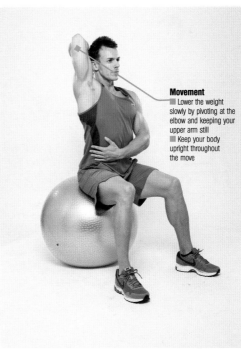

08

Dumb-bell overhead triceps extension

Target: triceps
This move encourages you to stabilise your body while working the long head of the triceps brachii for defined muscles.

Start position
■ Start with your torso upright and the weight above your head with your arm straight

Movement
■ Lower the weight slowly by pivoting at the elbow and keeping your upper arm still
■ Keep your body upright throughout the move

Dumb-bells & gym ball **I** Exercises

09

Two-arm dumb-bell kickback

Target: triceps, core

Work the triceps on both arms and challenge your core at the same time.

Start position
- Bend forwards at the hips and keep your back in its natural arch
- Start with your elbows bent at 90°

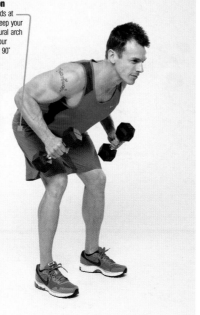

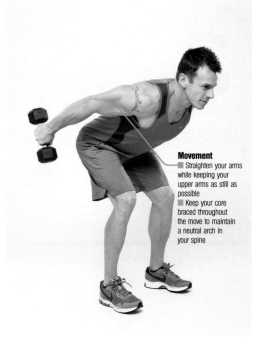

Movement
- Straighten your arms while keeping your upper arms as still as possible
- Keep your core braced throughout the move to maintain a neutral arch in your spine

10

Gym ball chair dip

Target: triceps, core

Increase the challenge to your triceps and core by placing your feet on a gym ball.

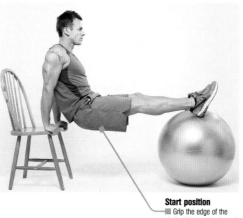

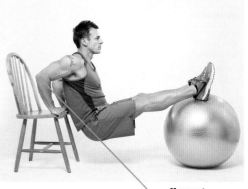

Start position
- Grip the edge of the chair with your hands and rest your heels on top of a gym ball
- Keep your feet together, your legs straight and your back upright

Movement
- Lower your body straight down, keeping your elbows pointing back, then press back up powerfully

Exercises **|** Dumb-bells & gym ball

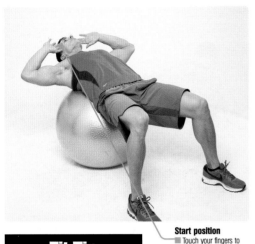

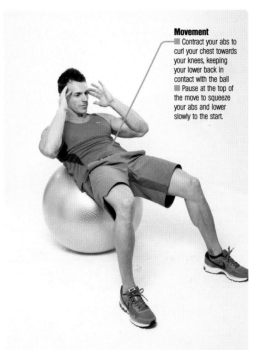

Movement
- Contract your abs to curl your chest towards your knees, keeping your lower back in contact with the ball
- Pause at the top of the move to squeeze your abs and lower slowly to the start.

11

Gym ball crunch

Target: abdominals

Using a gym ball increases your range of motion, giving your abdominal muscles a fuller workout while the instability challenges your core.

Start position
- Touch your fingers to your temples and lean as far back as you can on the ball

Fit Tip

Stay on the ball

Gym balls are great because they're wobbly. This forces your muscles, including your abs, to work harder to stabilise your body during any exercise than if you were on a solid surface.

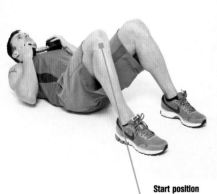

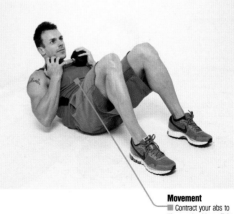

12

Dumb-bell crunch

Target: upper abdominals

Adding weight rather than doing more reps will have a better muscle-building effect on your abs so, if you find crunches easy, add resistance by using a dumb-bell.

Start position
- Keep your feet on the floor and your knees bent at 90˚ throughout the move
- Hold your head off the floor but keep your lower back in contact with the floor
- Hold the dumb-bell to your chest

Movement
- Contract your abs to lift your shoulders off the floor, pause at the top of the move to squeeze your abs, and lower slowly to the start

Dumb-bells & gym ball I **Exercises**

13

Gym ball oblique crunch

Target: obliques (side abs)
Hit your abs from the sides and get a broad range of motion by performing an oblique crunch on a gym ball.

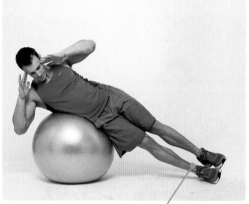

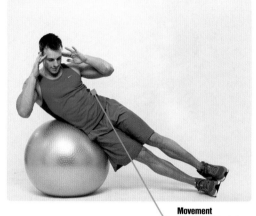

Start position
- Jam your feet against a support
- Lie sideways and curl your body around the ball

Movement
- Use your side abs to crunch up sideways, hold for a second at the top of the move, and lower under control

14

Gym ball side plank

Target: core
Plank exercises are great for developing core strength. Doing them on a gym ball makes them even more challenging.

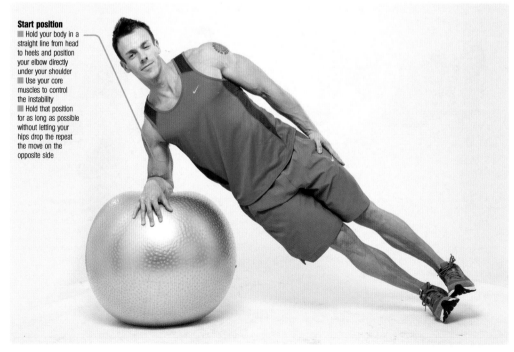

Start position
- Hold your body in a straight line from head to heels and position your elbow directly under your shoulder
- Use your core muscles to control the instability
- Hold that position for as long as possible without letting your hips drop the repeat the move on the opposite side

Exercises **I** Dumb-bells & gym ball

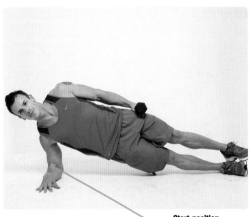

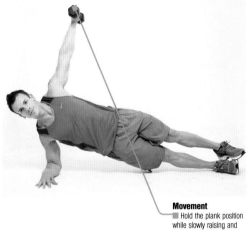

15

Side plank with lateral raise

Target: core, deltoids
Adding a lateral raise to a side plank increases the challenge to your core and improves your coordination.

Start position
■ Hold your body in a straight line from head to heels and position your elbow directly under the shoulder

Movement
■ Hold the plank position while slowly raising and lowering the weight
■ Use a light weight to maintain perfect form

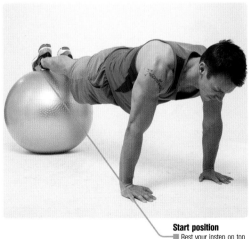

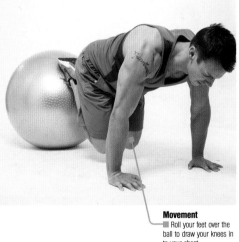

16

Gym ball jackknife

Target: upper and lower abdominals
The instability and range of motion involved in this move allow you to hit both your upper and lower abdominals.

Start position
■ Rest your instep on top of the ball with your body in a straight line and your hands directly beneath your shoulders

Movement
■ Roll your feet over the ball to draw your knees in to your chest
■ Try to avoid raising your backside as you move the ball

Dumb-bells & gym ball I Exercises

 17

Gym ball passing jackknife

Target: upper and lower abdominals
Using a gym ball encourages you to maintain perfect form throughout the move.

A

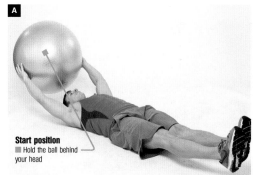

Start position
■ Hold the ball behind your head

B

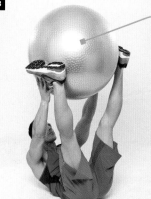

Movement
■ Keeping your arms and legs as straight as you can, pass the ball from hands to feet at the top of the move
■ Lower slowly with the ball clasped between your feet and return the ball to your hands on the next rep

C

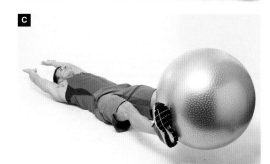

 18

Seated Russian twist

Target: obliques
Work your side abs and your core with this functional exercise that's good for sports that involve twisting moves.

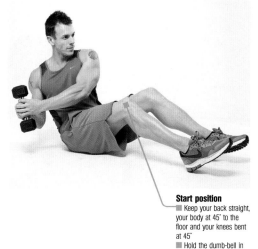

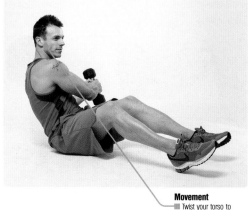

Start position
■ Keep your back straight, your body at 45˚ to the floor and your knees bent at 45˚
■ Hold the dumb-bell in both hands to one side of your body

Movement
■ Twist your torso to one side but keep looking straight ahead
■ Twist your torso to the opposite side, using your abs to control the momentum

Exercises **I** Dumb-bells & gym ball

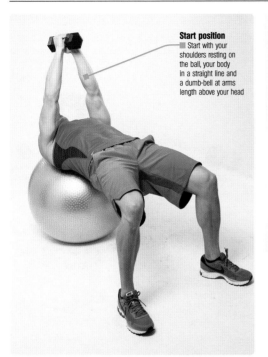

Start position
■ Start with your shoulders resting on the ball, your body in a straight line and a dumb-bell at arms length above your head

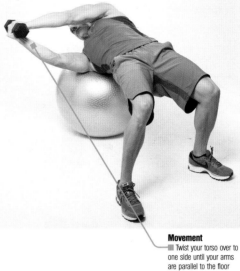

Movement
■ Twist your torso over to one side until your arms are parallel to the floor
■ Twist back to the opposite side, looking in the direction of the dumb-bell

19

Gym ball dumb-bell Russian twist

Target: core
Using a gym ball takes some of the strain off your lower back but still poses a challenge to your core muscles.

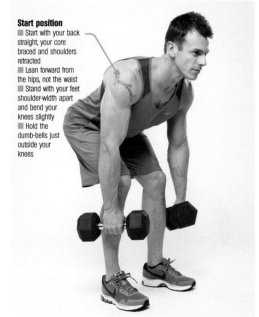

Start position
■ Start with your back straight, your core braced and shoulders retracted
■ Lean forward from the hips, not the waist
■ Stand with your feet shoulder-width apart and bend your knees slightly
■ Hold the dumb-bells just outside your knees

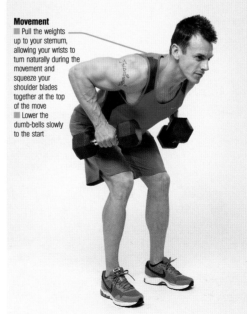

Movement
■ Pull the weights up to your sternum, allowing your wrists to turn naturally during the movement and squeeze your shoulder blades together at the top of the move
■ Lower the dumb-bells slowly to the start

20

Dumb-bell bent-over row

Target: traps, lats, rhomboids
Doing this classic back-building move with dumb-bells will give you balanced muscle development because it prevents your stronger side from taking more of the strain.

Dumb-bells & gym ball **I** Exercises

21

Bent-over flye

Target: upper back, shoulders

Get a strong upper back with this move that develops scapular retraction (the action of pulling your shoulder blades together).

Start position
■ Start with your back straight, your core braced and your shoulders retracted
■ Lean forward from the hips, not the waist
■ Stand with your feet shoulder width apart and bend your knees slightly
■ Hold the dumb-bells together just in front of your knees and keep a slight bend in your elbows

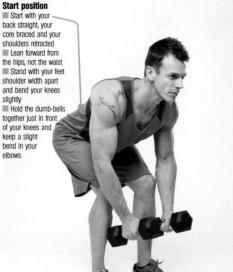

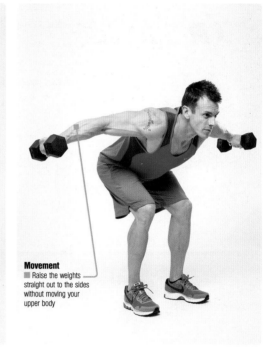

Movement
■ Raise the weights straight out to the sides without moving your upper body

22

Gym ball back extension

Target: lower back

Using a gym ball for this move gives you a broad range of motion. It's also a crucial move for balancing the training effect of doing crunches and for improving posture.

Start position
■ Wrap your body around the ball and jam your feet against a wall for support

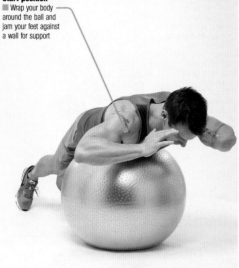

Movement
■ Lift your back until your body forms a straight line, but don't over-extend

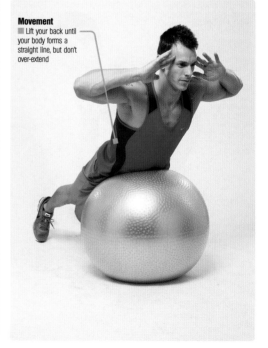

Exercises I Dumb-bells & gym ball

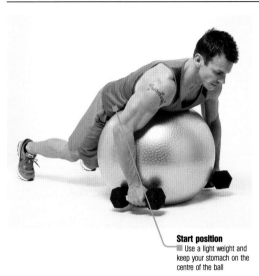

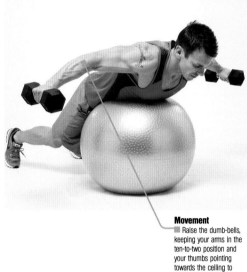

Start position
■ Use a light weight and keep your stomach on the centre of the ball

Movement
■ Raise the dumb-bells, keeping your arms in the ten-to-two position and your thumbs pointing towards the ceiling to activate your stabilising muscles
■ Pause at the top of the move and lower the weights slowly

23

Gym ball dumb-bell reverse flye

Target: back, shoulders, core
Chest and shoulder pressing moves work the front of your shoulder. This move will help you achieve balanced muscle gains because it works the back of your shoulders.

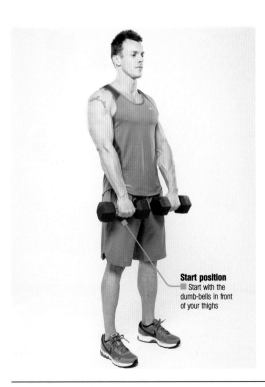

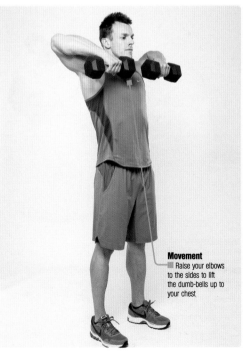

Start position
■ Start with the dumb-bells in front of your thighs

Movement
■ Raise your elbows to the sides to lift the dumb-bells up to your chest

24

Dumb-bell upright row

Target: upper traps, shoulders
Develop your upper back and shoulders while increasing your upright pulling strength.

Dumb-bells & gym ball **I** Exercises

25

Dumb-bell shrug

Target: upper traps

Add size to your upper back with this balanced move, which will also help stabilise your shoulder girdle and reduce your chances of sustaining a shoulder injury.

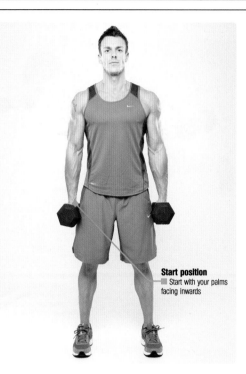

Start position
■ Start with your palms facing inwards

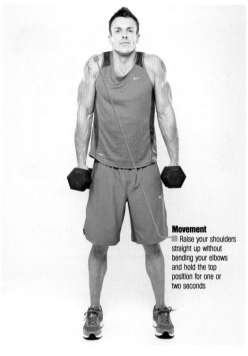

Movement
■ Raise your shoulders straight up without bending your elbows and hold the top position for one or two seconds

26

Gym ball dumb-bell press

Target: chest

Using dumb-bells for this classic chest exercise will give you a good range of movement, balanced muscle development and will recruit your glutes and core to stabilise the move.

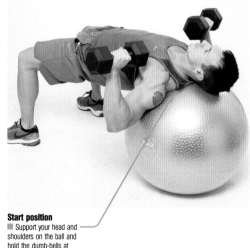

Movement
■ Press the weights up then lower slowly to the start

Start position
■ Support your head and shoulders on the ball and hold the dumb-bells at chest level
■ Brace your core and make sure that your body is straight form head to knees and your knees are bent at 90˚.

Exercises **I** Dumb-bells & gym ball

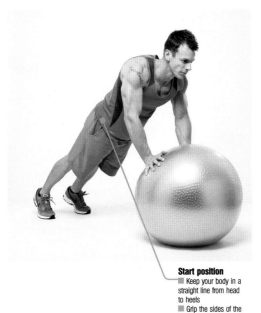

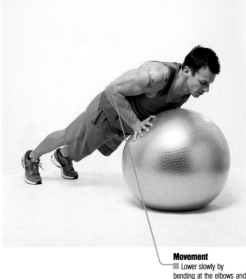

27

Gym ball press-up

Target: chest, triceps
Performing a press-up on a gym ball forces your chest muscles to control the movement, which will help you when you come to perform heavier pressing exercises.

Start position
■ Keep your body in a straight line from head to heels
■ Grip the sides of the ball roughly in line with your shoulders

Movement
■ Lower slowly by bending at the elbows and push back up powerfully

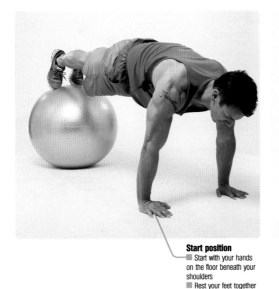

28

Gym ball decline press-up

Target: chest, shoulders, triceps, core
Resting your feet on top of a gym ball adds instability, which gives your core a good workout.

Start position
■ Start with your hands on the floor beneath your shoulders
■ Rest your feet together on top of the ball

Movement
■ Perform a press up but don't let your hips sag

Dumb-bells & gym ball I Exercises

33

Gym ball dumb-bell flye

Target: chest
This exercise primarily targets your pecs but also recruits your core and glutes to stabilise the move.

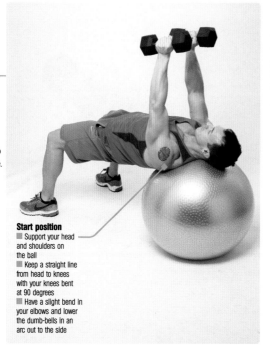

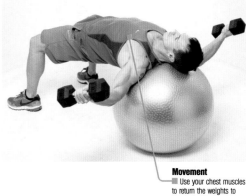

Movement
■ Use your chest muscles to return the weights to the start without arching your back

Start position
■ Support your head and shoulders on the ball
■ Keep a straight line from head to knees with your knees bent at 90 degrees
■ Have a slight bend in your elbows and lower the dumb-bells in an arc out to the side

34

Dumb-bell T press-up

Target: chest, shoulders, arms, core
Turn the press-up into an explosive move that works your body in more than one plane of motion.

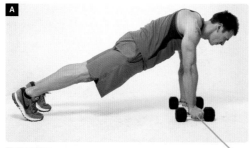

A

Start position
■ Grip the dumb bells with straight wrists and position them below your shoulders
■ Keep your body in a straight line and your elbows tucked in to your body
■ Keep your feet shoulder width apart and don't let your hips sag

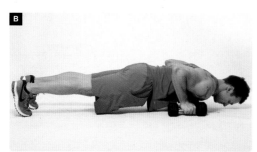

B

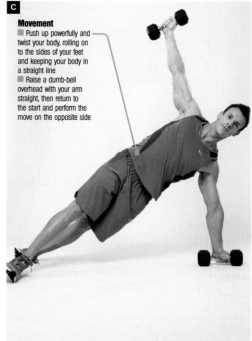

C

Movement
■ Push up powerfully and twist your body, rolling on to the sides of your feet and keeping your body in a straight line
■ Raise a dumb-bell overhead with your arm straight, then return to the start and perform the move on the opposite side

Exercises | Dumb-bells & gym ball

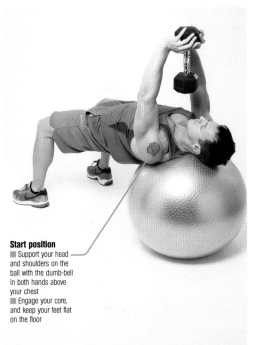

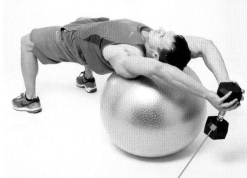

31

Gym ball dumb-bell pullover

Target: chest, lats, core
Use this single-joint move to hit multiple muscle groups.

Movement
■ Lower the weight slowly behind your head, keeping a slight bend in your elbows
■ Use your chest muscles to pull the weight back to the start but avoid arching your back to aid the move

Start position
■ Support your head and shoulders on the ball with the dumb-bell in both hands above your chest
■ Engage your core, and keep your feet flat on the floor

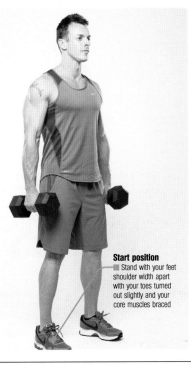

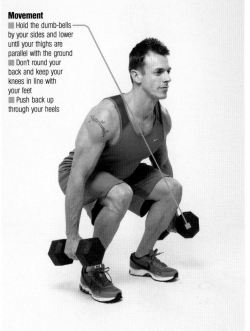

Movement
■ Hold the dumb-bells by your sides and lower until your thighs are parallel with the ground
■ Don't round your back and keep your knees in line with your feet
■ Push back up through your heels

32

Dumb-bell squat

Target: quads, glutes, hamstrings
Hit several major muscle groups at once with this must-do leg move.

Start position
■ Stand with your feet shoulder width apart with your toes turned out slightly and your core muscles braced

Dumb-bells & gym ball I Exercises

33

Dumb-bell sumo squat

Target: quads

By taking a wider stance you place more emphasis on the inside of your quads.

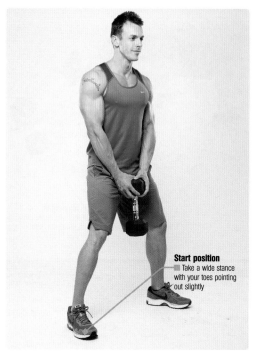

Start position
■ Take a wide stance with your toes pointing out slightly

Movement
■ Grip a dumb-bell with both hands and lower until your thighs are parallel to the floor
■ Keep your knees in line with your toes and keep your back upright

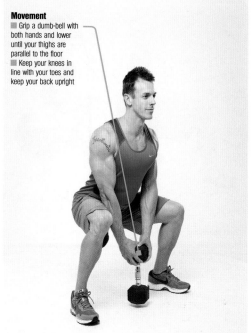

34

Dumb-bell gym ball wall squat

Target: quads

This is a great move if you're unused to doing squats because using a ball will engage your core and improve your coordination for this kind of movement.

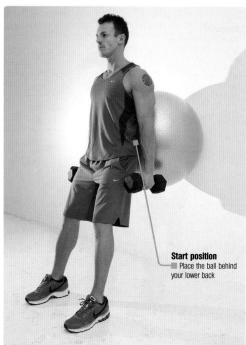

Start position
■ Place the ball behind your lower back

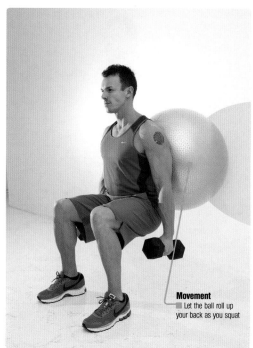

Movement
■ Let the ball roll up your back as you squat

Exercises | Dumb-bells & gym ball

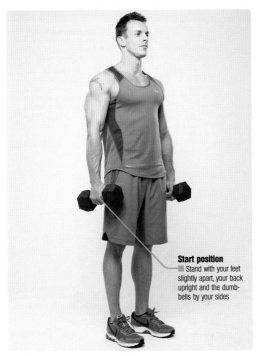

Start position
■ Stand with your feet slightly apart, your back upright and the dumb-bells by your sides

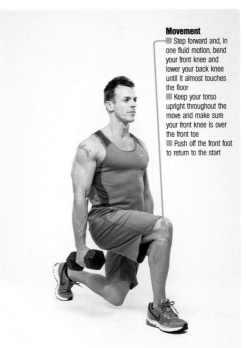

Movement
■ Step forward and, in one fluid motion, bend your front knee and lower your back knee until it almost touches the floor
■ Keep your torso upright throughout the move and make sure your front knee is over the front toe
■ Push off the front foot to return to the start

35

Dumb-bell lunge

Target: quads, hamstrings
Build muscle, increase your power and improve your coordination with this classic leg move.

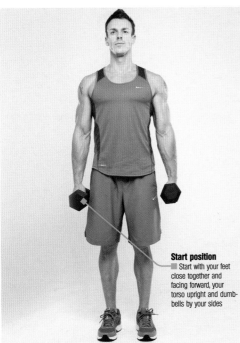

Start position
■ Start with your feet close together and facing forward, your torso upright and dumb-bells by your sides

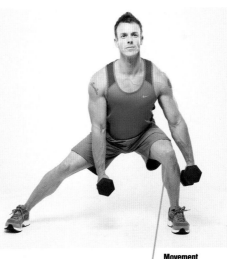

36

Dumb-bell side lunge

Target: adductors
Focus on your inner thighs to make sure you don't have any weak spots in your legs and improve your properioception – the body's ability to sense its movements.

Movement
■ Take a big step to the side, lowering onto your leading leg
■ Keep your torso upright throughout the move and your head facing forwards and your bent knee in line with your foot.

Dumb-bells & gym ball I Exercises

37

Dumb-bell reverse lunge

Target: quads, hamstrings

By stepping backwards instead of forwards you target your quads and hamstrings in a different way and increase the coordination challenge.

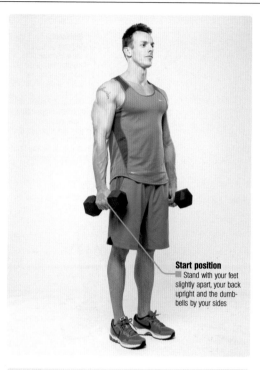

Start position
■ Stand with your feet slightly apart, your back upright and the dumb-bells by your sides

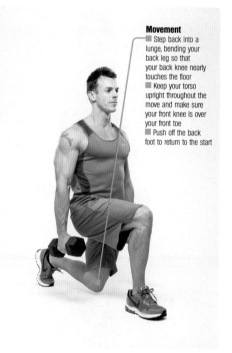

Movement
■ Step back into a lunge, bending your back leg so that your back knee nearly touches the floor
■ Keep your torso upright throughout the move and make sure your front knee is over your front toe
■ Push off the back foot to return to the start

38

Dumb-bell chair step-up

Target: quads, glutes

This exercise has real-life benefits because you do this move every day when you climb stairs.

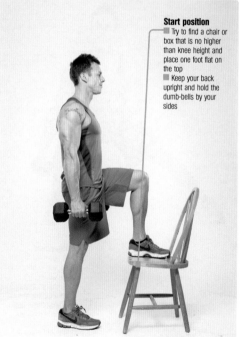

Start position
■ Try to find a chair or box that is no higher than knee height and place one foot flat on the top
■ Keep your back upright and hold the dumb-bells by your sides

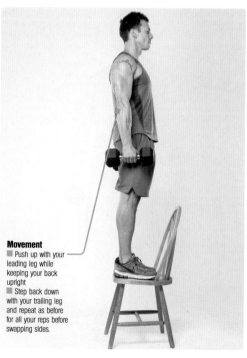

Movement
■ Push up with your leading leg while keeping your back upright
■ Step back down with your trailing leg and repeat as before for all your reps before swapping sides.

Exercises **|** Dumb-bells & gym ball

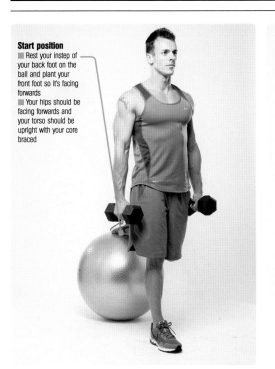

Start position
- ■ Rest your instep of your back foot on the ball and plant your front foot so it's facing forwards
- ■ Your hips should be facing forwards and your torso should be upright with your core braced

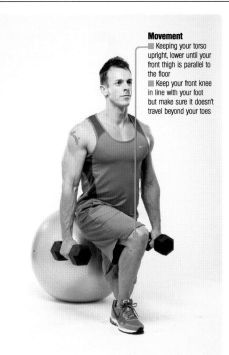

Movement
- ■ Keeping your torso upright, lower until your front thigh is parallel to the floor
- ■ Keep your front knee in line with your foot but make sure it doesn't travel beyond your toes

39

Gym ball dumb-bell Bulgarian split squat

Target: quads, glutes

Placing one foot on the ball deactivates that leg and places all the emphasis on your front leg.

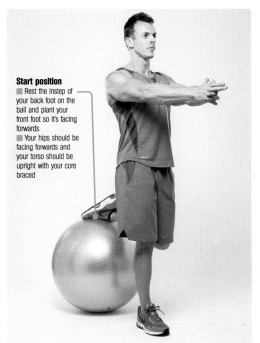

Start position
- ■ Rest the instep of your back foot on the ball and plant your front foot so it's facing forwards
- ■ Your hips should be facing forwards and your torso should be upright with your core braced

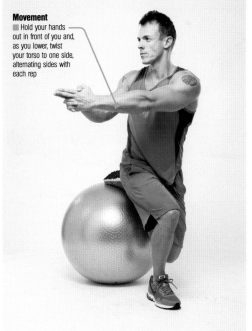

Movement
- ■ Hold your hands out in front of you and, as you lower, twist your torso to one side, alternating sides with each rep

40

Gym ball Bulgarian split squat with twist

Target: quads, glutes

Removing the dumb-bell but adding a twist makes the move more of a test of coordination and works your body in several planes at the same time.

Dumb-bells & gym ball I Exercises

41

Split dumb-bell Romanian deadlift

Target: hamstrings

Develop the backs of your legs but make sure you use perfect form to protect your back. This move has huge functional benefits because it's similar to the movements you make when bending down to pick something up.

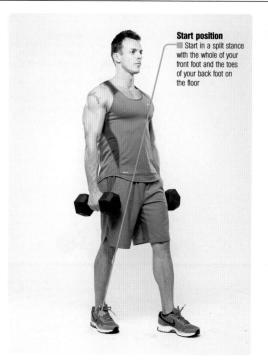

Start position
■ Start in a split stance with the whole of your front foot and the toes of your back foot on the floor

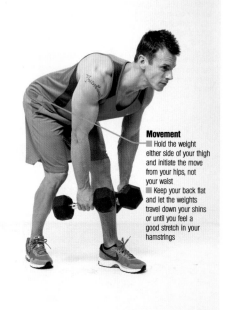

Movement
■ Hold the weight either side of your thigh and initiate the move from your hips, not your waist
■ Keep your back flat and let the weights travel down your shins or until you feel a good stretch in your hamstrings

42

Gym ball hamstring curl

Target: hamstrings

This move will develop your hamstrings while improving your stability in your hips and lower back.

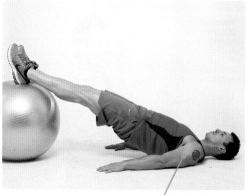

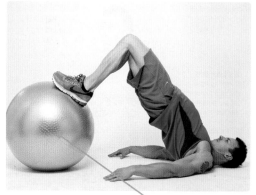

Start position
■ Rest your head and shoulders on the floor and keep your body in a straight line from shoulders to heels with your arms by your sides and your heels on top of the ball

Movement
■ Raise your hips and drag the ball towards your backside with your heels, keeping your body straight throughout the move
■ Pause at the top of the move and return slowly to the start

Exercises I Dumb-bells & gym ball

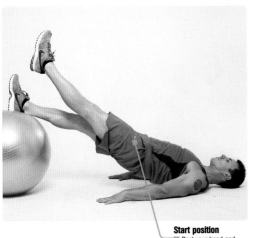

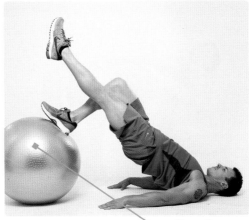

43

One-leg gym ball hamstring curl

Target:
Hamstrings
Doing the curl with one leg really gets your muscles working hard to control the wobble of the ball.

Start position
■ Rest your head and shoulders on the mat and keep your body in a straight line from shoulders to heels
■ Position your arms by your sides with one heel on top of the ball and the other leg raise slightly

Movement
■ Curl the ball towards your backside with your heel, pause and return to the start

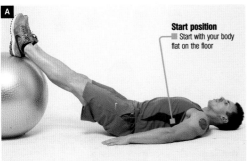

A

Start position
■ Start with your body flat on the floor

B

44

Gym ball hip raise and leg curl

Target:
hamstrings,
hip flexors
Starting the move with a hip raise works your hip flexors before targeting your hamstrings.

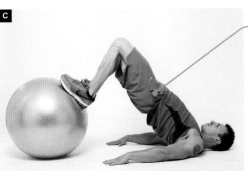

C

Movement
■ Raise your hips until your body is straight from shoulders to heels
■ Drag the ball towards your backside with your heels

Dumb-bells & gym ball I Exercises

45

Supine gym ball calf raise

Target: calves
This works your hard-to-target calves, forcing them to stabilise your entire body, which will help during bigger lifts.

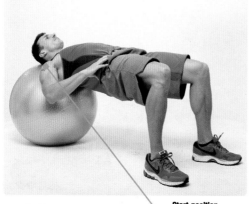

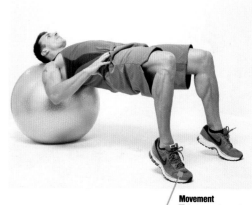

Fit Tip

Limit your reps

Increase muscle size by increasing the resistance rather than the number of reps. Try holding a dumb-bell on your chest during calf raises.

Start position
■ Rest your head and shoulders on the ball with your body in a straight line and your knees bent at 90 degrees

Movement
■ Push up onto your toes and hold for a two-count before lowering

46

Gym ball dumb-bell shoulder press

Target: deltoids
Using dumb-bells allows your arms to move in a natural arc and will give you balanced muscle development. The gym ball calls on your stabilising muscles to keep your torso steady throughout the move.

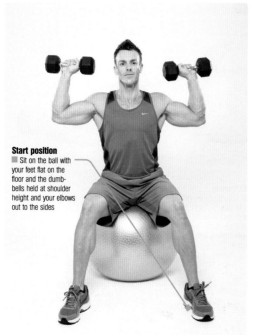

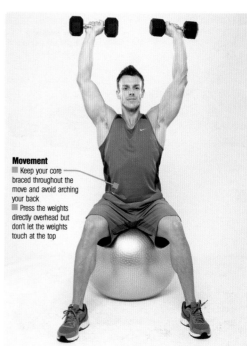

Start position
■ Sit on the ball with your feet flat on the floor and the dumb-bells held at shoulder height and your elbows out to the sides

Movement
■ Keep your core braced throughout the move and avoid arching your back
■ Press the weights directly overhead but don't let the weights touch at the top

Exercises **I** Dumb-bells & gym ball

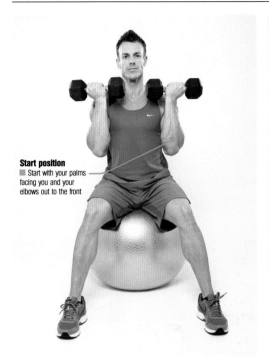

Start position
■ Start with your palms facing you and your elbows out to the front

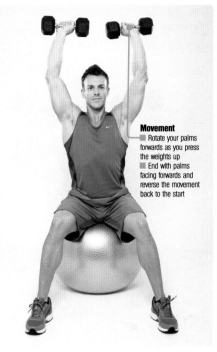

Movement
■ Rotate your palms forwards as you press the weights up
■ End with palms facing forwards and reverse the movement back to the start

47

Gym ball dumb-bell Arnold press

Target: deltoids
Introducing rotation to the move hits your deltoids from several angles in the same exercise.

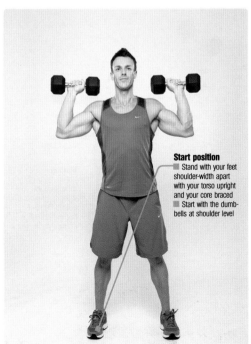

Start position
■ Stand with your feet shoulder-width apart with your torso upright and your core braced
■ Start with the dumb-bells at shoulder level

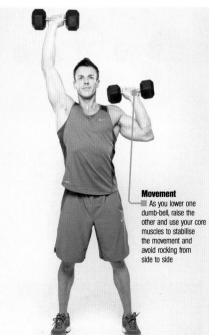

Movement
■ As you lower one dumb-bell, raise the other and use your core muscles to stabilise the movement and avoid rocking from side to side

48

Alternating dumb-bell shoulder press

Target: deltoids
Focusing on one shoulder at a time makes each side work as hard as possible and gives you balanced muscle growth.

Dumb-bells & gym ball I **Exercises**

49

Rotating squat press

Target: whole body
Add a squat and rotation to turn a shoulder move into a whole-body exercise.

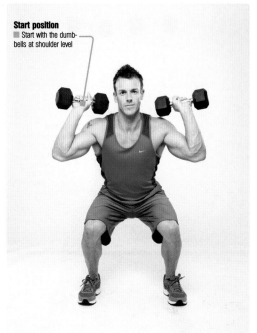

Start position
■ Start with the dumb-bells at shoulder level

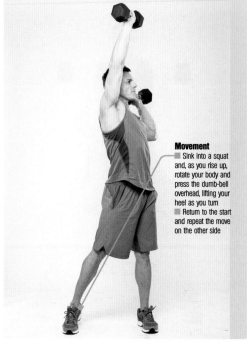

Movement
■ Sink into a squat and, as you rise up, rotate your body and press the dumb-bell overhead, lifting your heel as you turn
■ Return to the start and repeat the move on the other side

50

Alternating wide shoulder press

Target: deltoids
Hit your deltoids from a slightly different angle with this variation of the classic shoulder press.

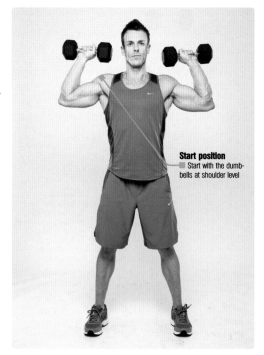

Start position
■ Start with the dumb-bells at shoulder level

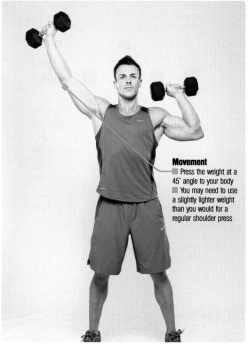

Movement
■ Press the weight at a 45° angle to your body
■ You may need to use a slightly lighter weight than you would for a regular shoulder press

Exercises | Dumb-bells & gym ball

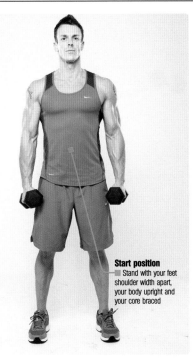

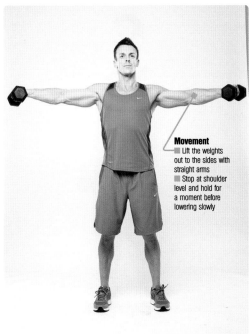

51

Lateral raise

Target: middle deltoid
Use a light weight and target your delts and upper traps to give yourself broad-looking shoulders.

Movement
■ Lift the weights out to the sides with straight arms
■ Stop at shoulder level and hold for a moment before lowering slowly

Start position
■ Stand with your feet shoulder width apart, your body upright and your core braced

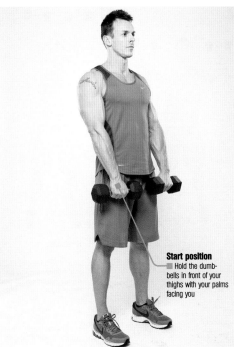

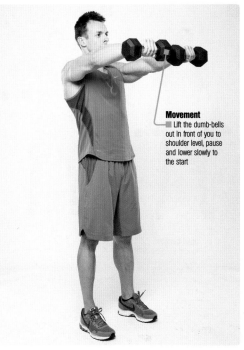

52

Front raise

Target: front deltoid
By raising the dumb-bells out in front of you, you place the stress on your front shoulders.

Movement
■ Lift the dumb-bells out in front of you to shoulder level, pause and lower slowly to the start

Start position
■ Hold the dumb-bells in front of your thighs with your palms facing you

Dumb-bells & gym ball I Exercises

53

Front/lateral raise

Target: middle, front deltoids

Alternate between front and lateral raises each time you lift the weight to hit your front and middle deltoids in the same move.

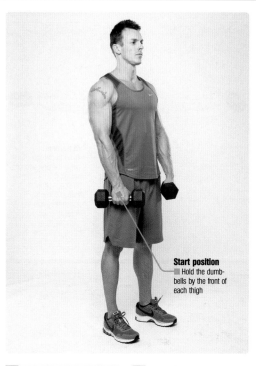

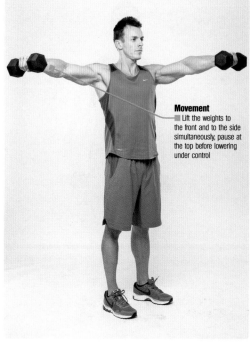

Start position
■ Hold the dumb-bells by the front of each thigh

Movement
■ Lift the weights to the front and to the side simultaneously, pause at the top before lowering under control

54

Cuban press

Target: rotator cuff

Strong and stable rotator cuffs are vital if you want to avoid shoulder injuries during heavy lifts. This move targets that often-neglected muscle.

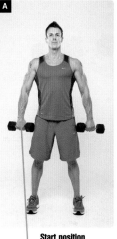

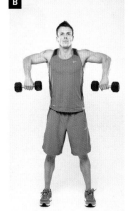

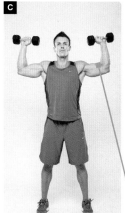

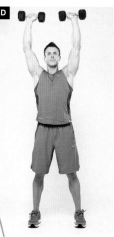

A **B** **C** **D**

Start position
■ Hold the dumb-bells out to your sides with your arms straight and your palms facing back

Movement
■ Lift your arms out to the sides until your elbows are bent at 90 degrees with the weights hanging straight down
■ Rotate your arms so your hands point up, keeping your upper arms horizontal
■ Press the weights directly overhead and reverse the movement back to the start

Exercises | Dumb-bells & gym ball

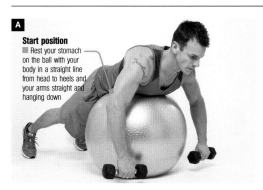

A

Start position
■ Rest your stomach on the ball with your body in a straight line from head to heels and your arms straight and hanging down

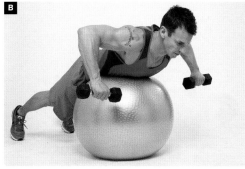

B

55

Gym ball lying Cuban press

Target: rotator cuffs
Using a ball encourages good posture because your body needs to stabilise the wobble.

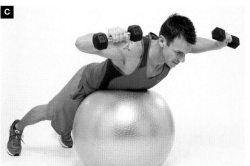

C

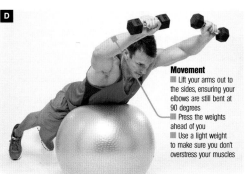

D

Movement
■ Lift your arms out to the sides, ensuring your elbows are still bent at 90 degrees
■ Press the weights ahead of you
■ Use a light weight to make sure you don't overstress your muscles

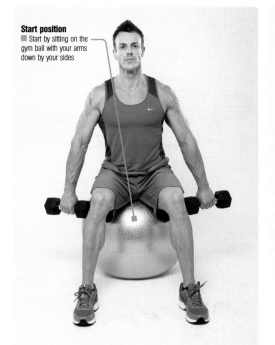

Start position
■ Start by sitting on the gym ball with your arms down by your sides

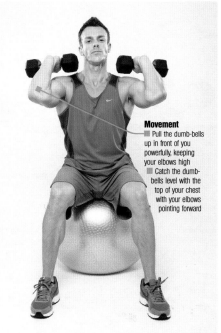

Movement
■ Pull the dumb-bells up in front of you powerfully, keeping your elbows high
■ Catch the dumb-bells level with the top of your chest with your elbows pointing forward

56

Gym ball dumb-bell cleans

Target: shoulders
Doing this explosive move with dumb-bells develops your shoulder stability, enabling you to pile on weight when you perform cleans with a barbell.

Dumb-bells & gym ball I Exercises

57

Internal dumb-bell rotation

Target: rotator cuff
Do this move as a warm-up before heavy shoulder exercises or at the end of a workout to develop your stabilising muscles.

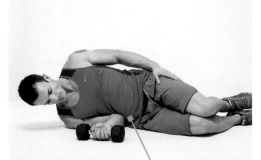

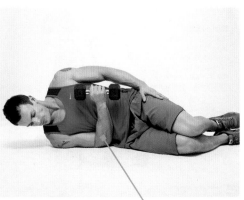

Fit Tip

Work your rotator cuffs

If you don't work on your rotator cuff you risk injuring your shoulders during big lifts such as snatches. Use a light weight and comparatively high reps to stabilise your shoulder joint.

Start position
■ Lie on your side with your knees bent for stability and your upper arm in line with your body and your elbow bent at 90°
■ Hold a light dumb-bell with an upturned palm

Movement
■ Rotate your arm so the dumb-bell points upwards with your elbow still at 90°

58

External dumb-bell rotation

Target: rotator cuff
Move your shoulder in the opposite direction to the internal rotation.

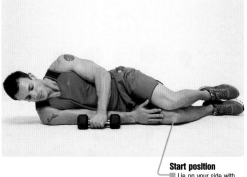

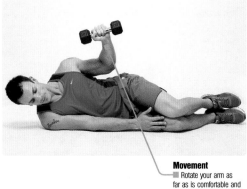

Start position
■ Lie on your side with your knees bent for stability
■ Hold a dumb-bell with your upper arm in line with your body and your elbow bent at 90°

Movement
■ Rotate your arm as far as is comfortable and return to the start

Exercises | Dumb-bells & gym ball

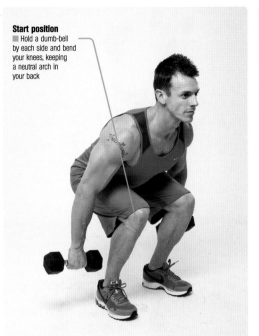

Start position
■ Hold a dumb-bell by each side and bend your knees, keeping a neutral arch in your back

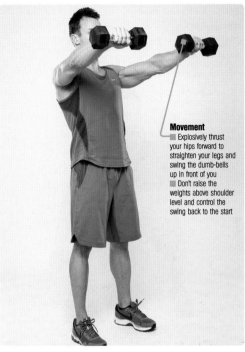

Movement
■ Explosively thrust your hips forward to straighten your legs and swing the dumb-bells up in front of you
■ Don't raise the weights above shoulder level and control the swing back to the start

59

Dumb-bell swing

Target: front shoulders, core, hamstrings
Work several muscle groups at once with this dynamic stability move which is good for power sports.

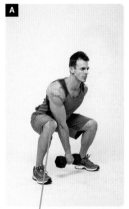

A

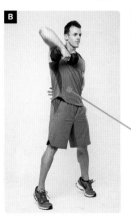

B

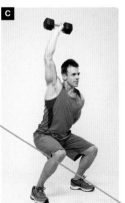

C

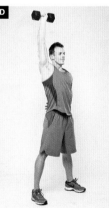

D

Start position
■ Start with your knees bent and hold one dumb-bell between your legs, keeping your shoulders square on

Movement
■ Straighten your legs and use the momentum to lift the weight up in front of you powerfully
■ Squat down beneath the weight to catch it with your arm straight
■ Stand up straight to complete the move

60

One-arm dumb-bell snatch

Target: whole body
This whole body move requires considerable coordination and develops power so it's great for sports such as football and rugby that require you to generate force in an upright position.

Dumb-bells & gym ball **|** Exercises

61

Dumb-bell woodchop

Target: whole body

This move is great for sports such as tennis that require twisting power because it connects your upper and lower body with one big rotational lift.

Start position
■ Start with your feet shoulder-width apart and your knees bent so that your thighs are almost parallel to the floor
■ Keep your back flat and twist your torso to the side, holding a dumb-bell in both hands on the outside of your thigh

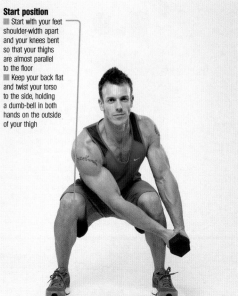

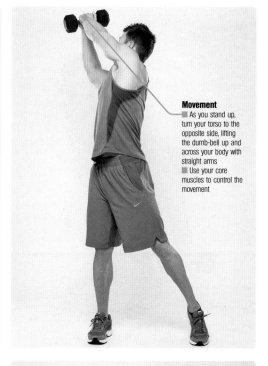

Movement
■ As you stand up, turn your torso to the opposite side, lifting the dumb-bell up and across your body with straight arms
■ Use your core muscles to control the movement

62

Woodchop lunge

Target: whole body

This move gets your body moving across three planes, which tests your balance and coordination and makes it a great move for sports conditioning.

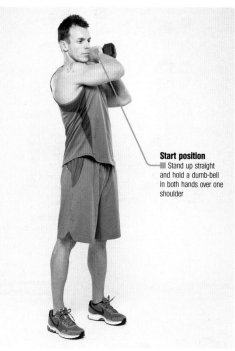

Start position
■ Stand up straight and hold a dumb-bell in both hands over one shoulder

Movement
■ Step forward into the lunge and chop the weight down and across your body
■ Make sure your front foot faces forward, your front knee is over your foot and your back is straight

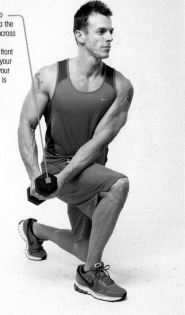

Exercises | Dumb-bells & gym ball

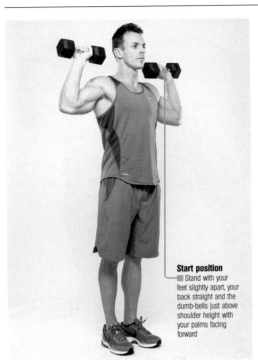

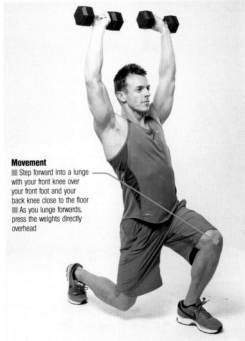

Movement
- Step forward into a lunge with your front knee over your front foot and your back knee close to the floor
- As you lunge forwards, press the weights directly overhead

Start position
- Stand with your feet slightly apart, your back straight and the dumb-bells just above shoulder height with your palms facing forward

63

Lunge to press

Target: whole body
Combine two compound moves to challenge every major muscle group and improve your hip and lower back stability.

A

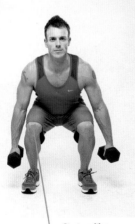

B

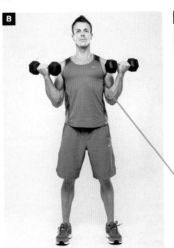

C

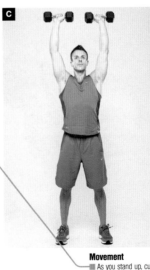

Start position
- Sink into a squat with your knees in line with your feet

Movement
- As you stand up, curl the dumb-bells up to your shoulders, keeping your elbows close to your sides
- Press the weights directly overhead and reverse the movement back to the start

64

Squat to curl to press

Target: whole body
Put three exercises together to make one fluid move that improves coordination and works your entire body without overloading any one joint.

Dumb-bells & gym ball I Exercises

65

Gym ball jackknife to press-up

Target: abs, hips, chest, triceps
This combination move teaches coordination of the core, hips and shoulders while giving you functional pushing strength.

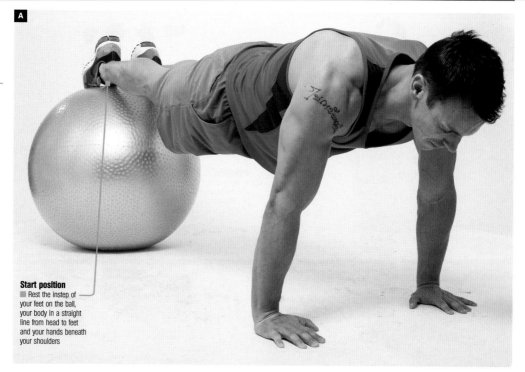

A

Start position
- Rest the instep of your feet on the ball, your body in a straight line from head to feet and your hands beneath your shoulders

B

C

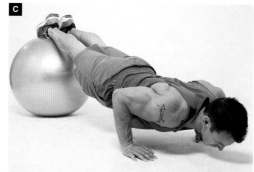

Movement
- Draw your knees up to your chest and return to the start
- Bend your elbows and lower your face to the floor to perform a press-up

Fit Tip

Make it hard on yourself
The press-up jackknife is a tough more but you can make it even more challenging by trying to do it with only one leg on the ball.

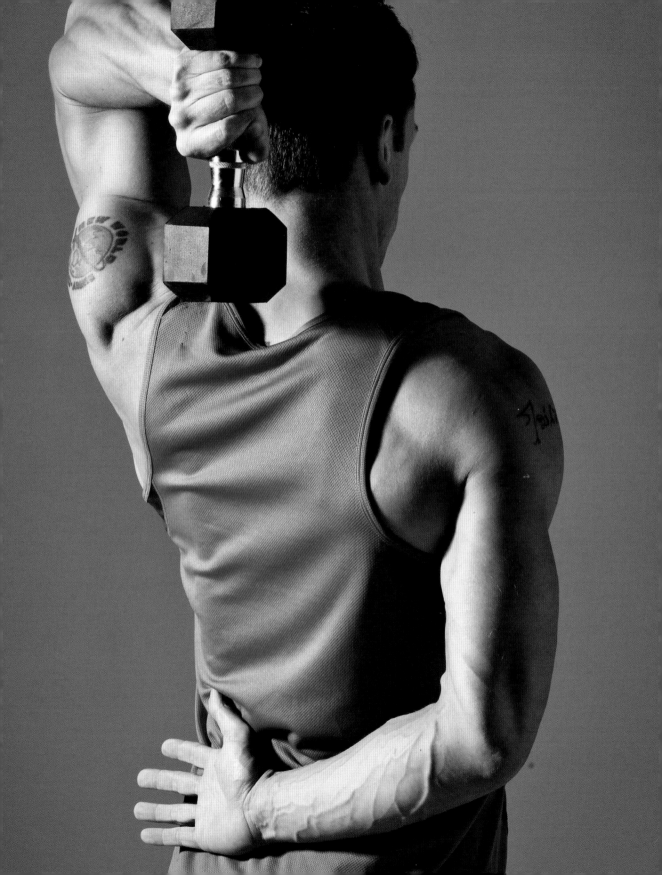

Dumb-bells & gym ball **I** Workouts

Full-body workout

Full-body workouts allow you to work a large range of muscle fibres in a relatively short space of time. This prompts your body to release a flood of growth hormones that will make your muscles get bigger and stronger. If you're new to training, they're useful because they get your muscles used to lifting weights without putting them under too much stress.

The downside of a full-body workout is that it's hard to fully exhaust your muscle fibres, so you may want to also do some more targeted sessions such as body-focus or post-exhaustion workouts, which we'll explore later.

Designing your workouts
Your full-body workouts need to be balanced. So, for every pushing motion you should do a pulling one, and you should spend as much time on your upper body as you do on your lower.

Stick to compound moves (the ones that work several muscle groups at once) because these will give you maximum muscle development for the time you have available.

Leave any abdominal moves to the end of your workout because you don't want them to be fatigued when you perform big moves such as squats and rows.

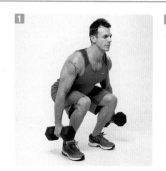

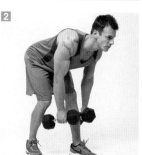

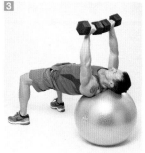

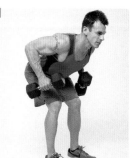

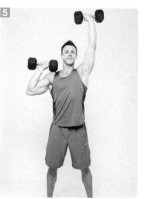

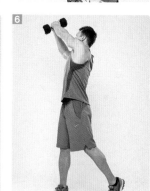

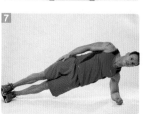

Full-body sample workout

1 Dumb-bell squat **I** **Sets:** 3 **Reps:** 10-12 **Page:** 67

2 Split dumb-bell Romanian deadlift
Sets: 2 **Reps:** 10 each side **Page:** 72

3 Gym ball dumb-bell press
Sets: 3 **Reps:** 10-12 **Page:** 64

4 Dumb-bell bent-over row **I** **Sets:** 3 **Reps:** 10-12 **Page:** 61

5 Alternating dumb-bell shoulder press
Sets: 2 **Reps:** 10 each side **Page:** 75

6 Dumb-bell woodchop
Sets: 2 **Reps:** 10 each side **Page:** 82

7 Side plank
Sets: 1 **Time:** hold for as long as possible **Page:** 30

Workouts | Dumb-bells & gym ball

Body focus workout

While full-body workouts let you work a big range of muscle groups, the advantage of body focus workouts is that you can completely fatigue the target muscles. You can then let them recover for a week while you train different body parts. It's a good way of being specific about how you put on muscle but the downside is that doing lots of single-joint exercises won't produce as big a growth hormone release as doing big compound moves. You also need to exercise frequently if you want to work every major muscle group once a week.

Designing your workout

The structure of your session is particularly important if you're doing a body focus routine because you want to train the target muscle hard but without overtraining or risking injury.

Start by doing light exercises that will warm up your joint before moving on to do the bigger muscle-building moves. You must then make sure you have fully fatigued the muscle by doing a single-joint move. Vary the exercises and angles you use to work that body part so that you get good and well balanced muscle growth.

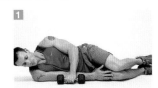

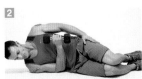

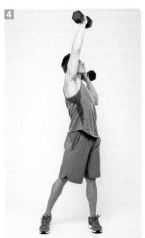

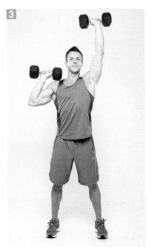

Body focus sample workout: shoulders

1 External dumb-bell rotation
Sets: 1 **Reps:** 15-20 **Page:** 80

2 Internal dumb-bell rotation
Sets: 1 **Reps:** 15-20 **Page:** 80

3 Alternating dumb-bell shoulder press
Sets: 2 **Reps:** 10 each side **Page:** 75

4 Rotating squat press | **Sets:** 2 **Reps:** 10 each side **Page:** 76

5 Gym ball Cuban press | **Sets:** 2 **Reps:** 10 **Page:** 79

6 Front/lateral raise | **Sets:** 2 **Reps:** 10 each side **Page:** 78

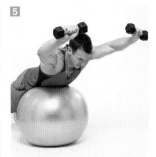

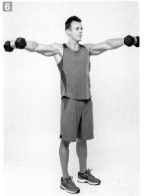

Dumb-bells & gym ball I Workouts

Core stability workout

As we identified in the no-kit workouts section, good core stability is absolutely essential if you want to lift heavy weights, be better at sport and stay injury free.

To recap, your core muscles are the ones around your midriff, including your abdominals and lower back, and their function is to provide a link between your upper and lower body. They're particularly important during whole-body moves, which need a strong core to transfer power between the upper and lower halves of your body. They're also called upon to stabilise your spine during dynamic and sporty movements.

A weak core will inhibit your ability to lift heavy weights in whole-body moves because you won't be able to transfer force from your lower to upper body. You may also be more likely to suffer from lower back and postural problems.

Developing your workout

To get a strong and stable core you need to attack the muscles from different angles and target the muscles at the sides and back of your midriff.

Start with moves that place the greatest weight on your core, such as compound lifts, and end with bodyweight exercises that won't risk injuring your tired muscles. Because this workout focuses on stability, you should complete a relatively high number of reps per set.

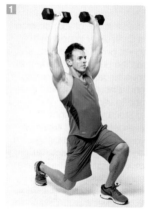

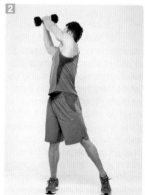

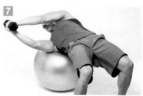

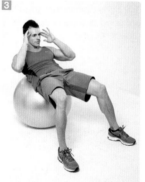

Core stability sample workout

1 Lunge to press I **Sets:** 2 **Reps:** 10-12 each side **Page:** 83

2 Dumb-bell woodchop
Sets: 2 **Reps:** 10-12 each side **Page:** 82

3 Gym ball crunch I **Sets:** 2 **Reps:** 15 **Page:** 57

4 Gym ball back extension I **Sets:** 2 **Reps:** 15 **Page:** 62

5 Gym ball oblique crunch
Sets: 2 **Reps:** 15 each side **Page:** 58

6 Two-point box I **Sets:** 2 **Reps:** 15 each side **Page:** 33

7 Gym ball dumb-bell Russian twist
Sets: 2 **Reps:** 15 each side **Page:** 61

8 Plank I **Sets:** 1 **Time:** Hold as long as possible **Page:** 29

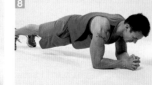

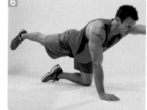

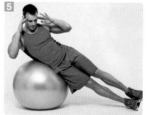

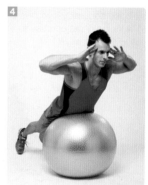

Circuit training workout

This is a great option if you're short of time or your main goal is fat loss. By doing different exercises back to back with no rest in between you keep your effort level high and force your heart to pump blood to different parts of your body, giving you both a cardiovascular and a muscle-building benefit. Be warned, this can be very tiring, so keep the weights light to avoid injury and fatiguing early. Circuits aren't the best way to build muscle but they will help you to look lean and defined.

Designing your workout

For circuits to be effective, you need to move from one exercise to the next as swiftly as possible so they work best when you can do all the moves in the workout with one item of kit.

Pick a group of exercises that target as many different muscle groups as possible and alternate between upper and lower body moves to make your heart work harder without experiencing excessive muscle fatigue.

Include a good mix of pushing, pulling, lunging, bending and rotational moves, to give your workout balance. You should also try to complete the reps quickly but without compromising good form. Once you have completed the circuit, rest for three minutes then do it all again. The fitter you become the more circuits you'll be able to complete.

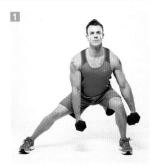

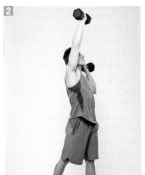

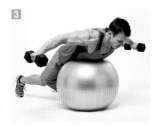

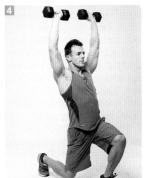

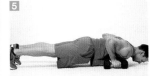

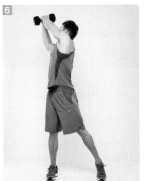

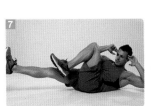

Circuit training sample workout

1 Dumb-bell side lunge
Sets: 1 **Reps:** 10 each side **Page:** 69

2 Rotating squat press | **Sets:** 1 **Reps:** 10 each side **Page:** 76

3 Gym ball dumb-bell reverse flye
Sets: 1 **Reps:** 10 **Page:** 63

4 Lunge to press | **Sets:** 1 **Reps:** 10 each side **Page:** 83

5 Dumb-bell T press-up | **Sets:** 1 **Reps:** 10 each side **Page:** 66

6 Dumb-bell woodchop
Sets: 1 **Reps:** 10 each side **Page:** 82

7 Bicycles | **Sets:** 1 **Reps:** 12 **Page:** 29

Dumb-bells & gym ball **I** Workouts

Explosive power workout

Explosive power workouts, also known as plyometric workouts, give you more than one of benefit. They help build muscle but also develop your power and coordination. During a plyometric move, you activate the muscle eccentrically as it's stretched out and pre-loaded, then you explode into the lift to contract the muscle concentrically, which shortens it.

This dynamic movement targets your fast-twitch muscle fibres, exhausting them quicker then a conventional workout but without having to add extra weight. The intensity will also push up your heart rate, burning extra calories and releasing muscle-building hormones into your body.

These types of workouts are popular with sportsmen because they can be used to develop fast, powerful movements and improve skills such as vertical leap.

Designing your workout

The intensity and force generated during explosive power workouts means that they carry a slightly higher injury risk. For that reason, you should perform fewer repetitions of each plyometric exercise than you would for a standard workout. For the plyometric moves, use either your bodyweight or a weight that's 30-40 per cent of your ten rep maximum for that exercise.

For each target body part, start by doing an activation move to warm up and stabilise your muscles. Then do the plyometric exercise before performing a single-joint move to exhaust the muscles.

The emphasis of these sessions is on speed and power, rather than developing endurance so make sure you rest for at least one minute between plyometric sets and at least two minutes between ployometric exercises.

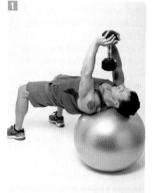
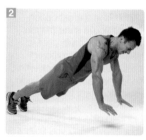
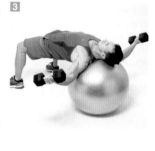
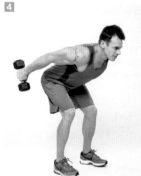
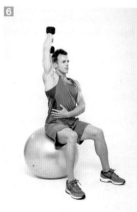
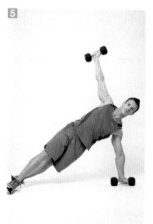

Explosive power sample workout:
chest and triceps

1 Gym ball dumb-bell pullover
Sets: 3 **Reps:** 10 **Page:** 67

2 Jumping press-up **I Sets:** 3 **Reps:** 8 **Page:** 36

3 Gym ball dumb-bell flye **I Sets:** 3 **Reps:** 10 **Page:** 66

4 Two-arm dumb-bell kickback **I Sets:** 3 **Reps:** 10 **Page:** 56

5 Dumb-bell T press-up
Sets: 2 **Reps:** 8 each side **Page:** 66

6 Dumb-bell overhead triceps extension
Sets: 2 **Reps:** 10 each side **Page:** 55

Superset workout

Supersets are a great time-saving option. Because you do two exercises back to back before resting, you dramatically reduce your workout time.

You can pair any two exercises to form a superset but the most popular option is to create 'antagonistic supersets', where the two moves work opposing body parts. An example would be to perform a gym ball dumb-bell press (which works your chest) then go straight into a dumb-bell bent-over row (which works your back). The advantage of antagonistic supersets is that they give one body part a chance to rest while the opposing muscle group is working, which leads to balanced muscle development. Other options include non-competing supersets, which target unrelated muscle groups such as pairing a lower-body move with an upper-body one, and post-exhaustion supersets, where you do a multi-joint move followed by a single-joint move targeting the same body part.

Designing your workout

For each exercise in this antagonistic superset workout, find one that works its polar opposite, so if you do one exercise that targets your quads do another that targets your hamstrings. Biceps exercises should be paired with triceps moves, and so on. After each superset, rest for two minutes and repeat.

1 Superset A

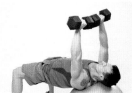

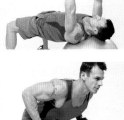

2 Superset B

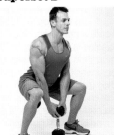

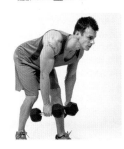

3 Superset C

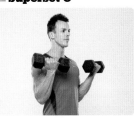

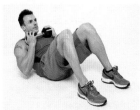

4 Superset D

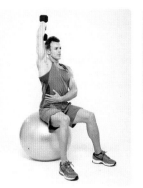

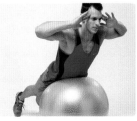

Superset sample workout

1 Superset A | Gym ball dumb-bell press | Dumb-bell bent-over row | **Sets:** 3 **Reps:** 10-12 **Pages:** 64, 61

2 Superset B | Dumb-bell sumo squat | Split dumb-bell Romanian deadlift | **Sets:** 3 **Reps:** 10-12 **Pages:** 68, 72

3 Superset C | Dumb-bell curl | Dumb-bell overhead triceps extension | **Sets:** 3 **Reps:** 10-12 **Pages:** 52, 55

4 Superset D | Dumb-bell crunch | Gym ball back extension | **Sets:** 3 **Reps:** 10-12 **Pages:** 57, 62

Dumb-bells & gym ball I **Workouts**

Body part split workout

As you become more advanced, you may find that you're unable to sufficiently fatigue your muscles in a full-body routine. If that's the case, you should consider doing a split routine where you do a different thing in each session of the week. The most popular form of split routine is a body part split where you train two body parts in a single session.

An example of this would be to train your chest and triceps in your first workout of the week, your shoulders and biceps in the second, your legs and back in the third and you abs and core in the fourth. This system lets you hit every body part hard once a week without having to go to the gym every day.

Designing your workout

Once you've decided on which two body parts you're going to work, do a move that works one of these body parts then alternate between the two body parts. So, for example, if you're going to work your shoulders and biceps you could start with a dumb-bell Arnold press, which works your shoulders and follow that with biceps curls, which work your biceps. To fully develop the body part, make sure you include a range of exercises that hit the target muscle groups from a variety of angles.

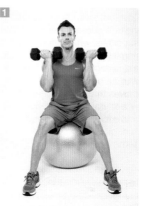

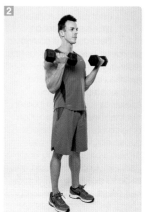

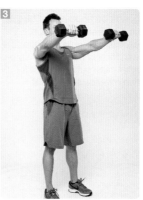

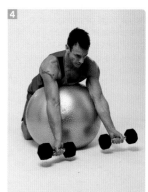

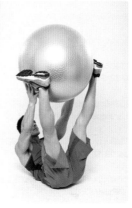

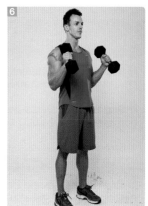

Body part split sample workout:
shoulders and biceps

1 Gym ball dumb-bell Arnold press
Sets: 3 **Reps:** 10-12 **Page:** 75

2 Dumb-bell curl I **Sets:** 3 **Reps:** 10-12 **Page:** 52

3 Front raise I **Sets:** 3 **Reps:** 10-12 **Page:** 77

4 Gym ball dumb-bell preacher curl
Sets: 2 **Reps:** 10 each side **Page:** 53

5 Gym ball passing jackknife I **Sets:** 3 **Reps:** 10-12 **Page:** 60

6 Hammer curl I **Sets:** 3 **Reps:** 10-12 **Page:** 54

Workouts | Dumb-bells & gym ball

Upper/lower body split workout

Another popular way of arranging a split routine is to do an upper/lower split, where you alternate between sessions made up entirely of upper or lower body moves.

This type of workout is simple to create so you don't have to spend lots of time planning your sessions. They also suit people who can't fit in many sessions per week because you only have to do two sessions a week to make sure you've worked every major muscle group. You will, however, need to do more than two sessions a week if you want to see the best benefits.

Designing your workout

If you're doing a lower-body day, all your exercises should target your lower body. You still need to make sure your routine is balanced, so include moves that work your glutes, quads, hamstrings and calves, and make sure you hit them from different angles.

Start with the biggest muscles such as your quads and hamstrings, then do calves moves.

If you're doing an upper-body workout, the same principles apply so you'd do chest, back and shoulders moves before targeting the smaller muscles of your biceps, triceps and forearms.

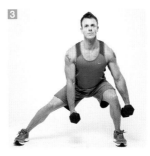
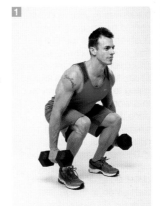
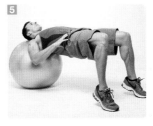
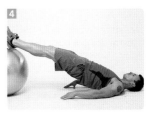
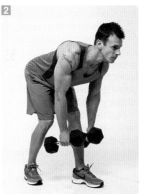
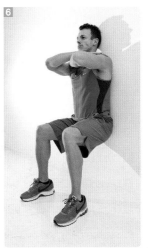

Upper/lower body split sample workout: lower body

1 Dumb-bell squat | **Sets:** 3 **Reps:** 10-12 **Page:** 67

2 Split dumb-bell Romanian deadlift
Sets: 2 **Reps:** 10 each side **Page:** 72

3 Dumb-bell side lunge | **Sets:** 2 **Reps:** 10 each side **Page:** 69

4 Gym ball hip raise leg curl | **Sets:** 3 **Reps:** 10-12 **Page:** 73

5 Supine gym ball calf raise | **Sets:** 3 **Reps:** 10-12 **Page:** 74

6 Wall squat
Sets: 1 **Time:** hold for as long as possible **Page:** 39

Dumb-bells & gym ball I Workouts

Push/pull split workout

A push/pull split routine is similar to an upper lower/body one in that you do two types of workout. In this case, you alternate between workouts involving pushing moves and workouts involving pulling moves.

This way of splitting workouts can be attractive for people who do sports that involve a lot of pushing movements, such as rugby. You still, however, need to do an equal amount of pulling moves to make sure you get balanced muscle development.

Designing your workout
If you're doing a push day, all the moves in your workout should be pushing moves. Pushing moves are ones that work your chest, quads, shoulders, triceps and calves. Aim to make your workout balanced, so include moves that work all of those body parts and use different exercises and angles in different push sessions.

Do moves that target your big muscles such as your chest, quads and shoulders then go on to the smaller muscles of your triceps and calves. If you're doing a pulling workout, the same rules apply, so you'd include moves that target your back, hamstrings, biceps and abs.

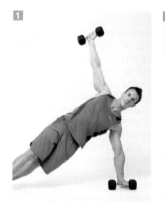

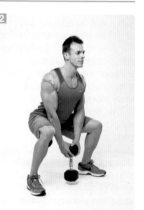

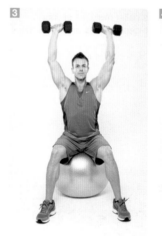

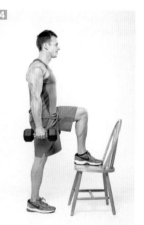

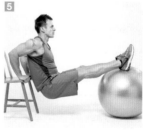

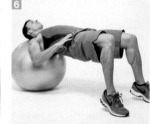

Push/pull split sample workout: push session

1 Dumb-bell T press-up I **Sets:** 2 **Reps:** 10 each side **Page:** 66

2 Dumb-bell sumo squat I **Sets:** 3 **Reps:** 10-12 **Page:** 68

3 Gym ball shoulder press I **Sets:** 3 **Reps:** 10-12 **Page:** 75

4 Dumb-bell step-up I **Sets:** 2 **Reps:** 10 each side **Page:** 70

5 Gym ball chair dip I **Sets:** 3 **Reps:** 10-12 **Page:** 56

6 Supine gym ball calf raise I **Sets:** 3 **Reps:** 10-12 **Page:** 74

Workouts | Dumb-bells & gym ball

Post-exhaustion workout

Weight training exercises can be divided into two main categories – compound moves and isolation moves. Compound exercises use several muscle groups at once while isolation exercises target one muscle group on its own. Post-exhaustion training involves pairing a compound move with an isolation one.

The theory is that you do a big muscle move to get yourself pumped by moving heavy weights. When you move onto the lighter weight isolation move you completely fatigue the target muscle. This is good for muscle growth because you exhaust a high number of muscle fibres. Your body then repairs those fibres to become bigger and stronger than they were before.

Designing your workout

If you're training your chest, you would start by doing your sets of a chest press, for example, which works your chest, triceps and shoulders. You could then move on to doing dumb-bell flyes, which focus on your chest.

You should avoid doing the isolation move first because this may fatigue your target muscle, which will be too tired to lift the heavy weight of a compound move. This increases the strain on your smaller supporting muscles, which may get injured as a result.

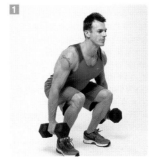
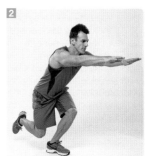
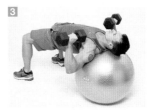
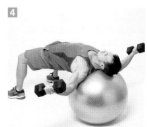
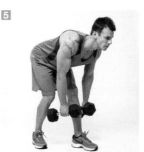
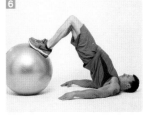
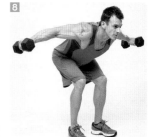
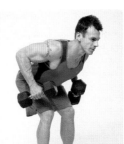

Post-exhaustion sample workout

1 Dumb-bell squat | **Sets:** 3 **Reps:** 10 **Page:** 67

2 Single-leg squat | **Sets:** 2 **Reps:** 10 each side **Page:** 38

3 Gym ball dumb-bell press | **Sets:** 3 **Reps:** 10 **Page:** 64

4 Gym ball dumb-bell flye | **Sets:** 3 **Reps:** 12 **Page:** 66

5 Split dumb-bell Romanian deadlift
Sets: 2 **Reps:** 10 each side **Page:** 72

6 Gym ball hamstring curl | **Sets:** 3 **Reps:** 12 **Page:** 72

7 Dumb-bell bent-over row | **Sets:** 3 **Reps:** 10 **Page:** 61

8 Bent-over flye | **Sets:** 3 **Reps:** 12 **Page:** 62

Dumb-bells & gym ball I Workouts

Drop set workout

Drop sets are a way of increasing the number of reps you perform of an exercise. Once you reach failure on your final set of an exercise, immediately reduce the weight and do as many reps as you can with that weight. Once you reach failure again, drop the weight once more and continue that process.

The intense nature of this system ramps up the muscle-building effect so use them to iron out weak muscle links. To do them effectively try to minimise the time between reaching failure and starting the new weight, so you don't get a chance to recover.

Designing your workout

Drop sets are a demanding technique so use them sparingly. Make sure that you

only do them on the final set of the final exercise of a body part because they completely exhaust the muscle involved. If you tried to do more exercises for that body part you would struggle to maintain perfect form.

For the same reason, you should only perform one or two drop sets per workout. Do more and you risk overtraining. You can use as many drops as you like, provided you maintain strict form. Make sure you drop the weight at increments that have a positive but not too dramatic an effect on how many reps you can perform. Dropping the weight by 20 per cent is a good place to start. If you halve the weight you won't take full advantage of the technique's muscle-building potential.

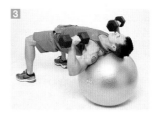

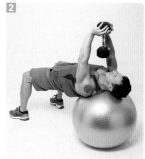

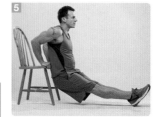

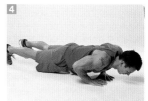

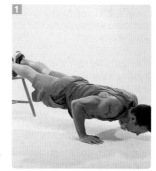

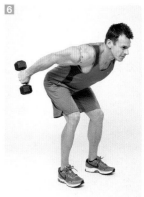

Drop set sample workout:
chest and triceps

1 Decline press-up I **Sets:** 2 **Reps:** 10 **Page:** 37

2 Gym ball dumb-bell pullover
Sets: 3 **Reps:** 10-12 **Page:** 67

3 Gym ball dumb-bell press
Sets: 3 (last set drop set) **Reps:** 10-12 **Page:** 64

4 Diamond press-up I **Sets:** 3 **Reps:** 10-12 **Page:** 35

5 Chair dip I **Sets:** 3 **Reps:** 10-12 **Page:** 26

6 Two-arm dumb-bell kickback
Sets: 3 (last set drop set) **Reps:** 10-12 **Page:** 56

Workouts **| Dumb-bells & gym ball**

Back-off set workout

These workouts typically involve doing between 2-4 sets of low reps with a heavy weight of an exercise before dropping the weight significantly for a final set where you do as many reps as possible.

The reason this is effective is because the nerves that stimulate your muscles are primed for action by the heavy sets, allowing you to perform better in the final set than you would had you attempted that set before the heavy sets. This increased capacity sparks new muscle growth.

Designing your workouts

In order for a back-off set to be effective, it has to be a move that you can do using heavy weights and one that you can control how much weight you're lifting. That's why big compound moves such as dumb-bell squats, rather than stability or bodyweight exercises, work most effectively.

You'll get best results by activating the target muscle group before working it again in a back off exercise. You'll also get a bigger muscle-building effect when you do your initial sets of the back-off exercise with low reps. But if your dumb-bells don't go over 10kg you might not be able to fatigue your muscle that quickly so you may have to do more reps.

For the back-off set, drop the weight by 40 per cent and do as many reps as you can with perfect form. If, for example, you ordinarily lift 10kg each side in a gym ball dumb-bell Arnold press, reduce this to 6kg per side for the back-off set.

Aim to perform the reps of a back-off set faster than you would during a regular set to develop your explosive power and your strength. This way of working out can be draining so only use it sparingly. Do it for one week as part of a six-to-eight week programme.

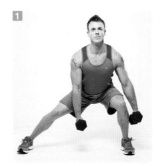

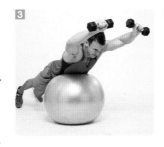

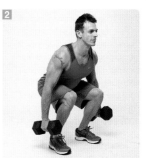

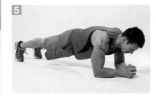

Back-off set sample workout:
legs, shoulders and core

1 Dumb-bell side lunge | **Sets: 2 Reps:** 10 each side **Page:** 69

2 Dumb-bell squat | **Sets:** 3 (+1 back-off set)
Reps: 10 (+ as many as you can in back-off set) **Page:** 67

3 Cuban press | **Sets:** 3 **Reps:** 10 **Page:** 79

4 Gym ball dumb-bell Arnold press | **Sets:** 3 (+1 back-off set) **Reps:** 10 (+ as many as you can in back-off set) **Page:** 75

5 Plank | **Sets:** 3 **Time:** 30 seconds **Page:** 29

6 Dumb-bell woodchop | **Sets:** 3 (+1 back-off set)
Reps: 10 (+ as many as you can in back-off set) **Page:** 82

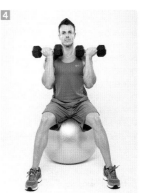

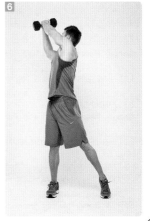

Dumb-bells & gym ball I Workouts

Pyramid workout

To grow your muscles you need to exhaust them so they repair to be stronger than they were before. The more fibres you exhaust, the greater your muscle growth. One way of maximising the number of fibres you stimulate is to do a pyramid workout.

Essentially, pyramid workouts involve increasing the weight that you lift with each set of an exercise while reducing the number of reps you perform. This is good because there's no such thing as a slightly activated muscle fibre – they are either engaged or not. By taking a muscle through an increasing range of weight while reducing the reps, you target each category of fibres in turn, completely exhausting the whole muscle.

Designing your workout
Doing a whole workout of pyramid exercises would take a long time and could

be counter productive, overtraining the muscle and sending the body into a destructive metabolism. Instead, strategically inserting pyramid sets into a workout will give you all the benefits of this method.

There is more than one way of performing a pyramid workout. You could start with a conventional muscle growth rep count, such as 12, and reduce the number of reps you do by two each set until you get to six reps. You can also do a reverse pyramid by starting with low reps and ending with a high rep count.

You can adjust your rep counts depending on what you want to achieve. If your focus is on strength, start with fewer reps and go down to as little as one rep for a set. You can also reduce your reps before gradually increasing them to finish with the same number of reps you completed for your first set.

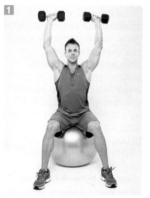
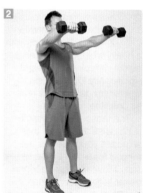

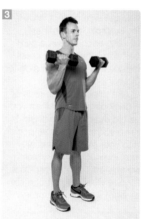
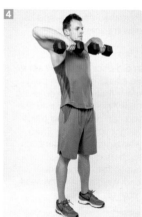

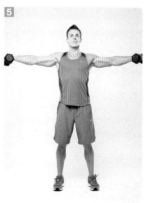
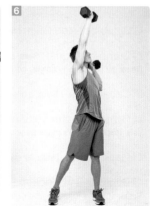

Pyramid sample workout:
shoulders and arms

1 Gym ball dumb-bell shoulder press
Sets: 4 Reps: Pyramid 12/10/8/6 **Page: 74**

2 Front raise I **Sets: 3 Reps:** 10-12 **Page: 77**

3 Dumb-bell curl
Sets: 2 Reps: 10 each side **Page: 52**

4 Dumb-bell upright row I **Sets: 3 Reps:** 10-12 **Page: 63**

5 Lateral raise I **Sets: 3 Reps:** 10-12 **Page: 77**

6 Rotating squat press
Sets: 4 Reps: Reverse pyramid 6/8/10/12 **Page: 76**

Workouts I Dumb-bells & gym ball

Wave-loading workout

There are a number of ways that you can do a wave-loading session but, essentially, they all involve lifting a weight for a set then cutting the reps but upping the weight for the next set. From here you can either go back to the original weight and perform as many reps as you can or reduce the reps and up the weight for another set before repeating that sequence of three sets.

Whatever way you decide to arrange your wave-loading workout, they teach your muscles to lift more weight in a single rep so they're a good tool to use if you're struggling to increase your maximum lift in a particular exercise.

Designing your workout
Wave-loading works well in split routines because you can activate the body part with a stability move before wave-loading for the strength move and fully exhausting the target muscle in an isolation move.

One option for wave-loading moves is to find your five repetition maximum for an exercise then do four reps. Rest for three minutes, increase the weight by five per cent then do three reps. Rest for three minutes, increase the weight by five per cent and do two reps. Rest for three minutes and repeat that sequence.

An alternative, and the one outlined in the sample workout on this page, is to do a normal set of eight reps then rest for two minutes before loading extra weight onto your dumb-bells for a shorter set of four reps. Another rest of two minutes is followed by a final set in which you go back to the original weight and crank out as many reps as possible, taking you past eight reps.

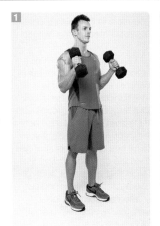
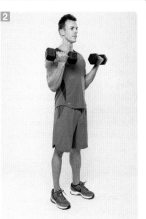
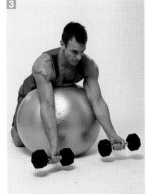
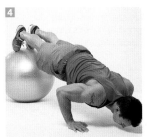
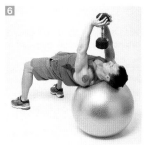
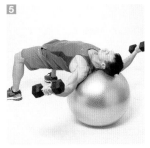

Wave loading sample workout:
chest and biceps

1 Hammer curl I **Sets: 3 Reps: 10-12 Page: 54**

2 Dumb-bell curl
Sets: 3 Reps: (wave loader) 8, 4, 8+ Page: 52

3 Gym ball dumb-bell preacher curl
Sets: 3 Reps: 10-12 Page: 53

4 Gym ball press-up I **Sets: 3 Reps: 10-12 Page: 65**

5 Gym ball dumb-bell flye
Sets: 3 Reps: (wave loader) 8, 4, 8+ Page: 66

6 Dumb-bell pull-over I **Sets: 3 Reps: 10-12 Page: 67**

Dumb-bells & gym ball I *Workouts*

Unilateral workout

When you lift a weight with both sides of your body, your stronger side will work harder in an effort to take the strain off your weaker side. If you continue to do lifts that work both sides of your body simultaneously, you may end up with unbalanced muscles.

The solution is to do unilateral workouts, which involve working one side of your body at a time. Doing that will force both sides of your body to work equally hard, resulting in equal muscle growth, which will make you look better and reduce your chances of getting injured. Unilateral moves are also good at developing your stabilising muscles because

you have to completely control the movement of the weight.

Designing your workout

Unilateral workouts can be used to address muscle imbalances, so do exercises that target muscle groups you think aren't balanced on both sides of your body. So, if you think one shoulder is stronger than the other, do moves that target that body part, such as alternating shoulder presses.

You can combine a unilateral workout with another workout style such as an explosive workout where you only do one-sided explosive moves. The workout sample on this page is an example of a whole-body unilateral workout.

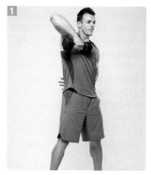

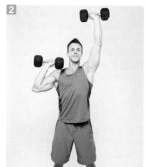

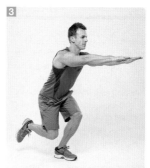

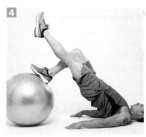

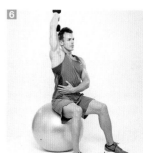

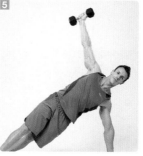

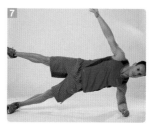

Unilateral sample workout

1 One-arm dumb-bell snatch I **Sets:** 2
Reps: 10 each side **Page:** 81

2 Alternating dumb-bell shoulder press I **Sets:** 2
Reps: 10 each side **Page:** 75

3 Single-leg squat I **Sets:** 2 **Reps:** 10 each side **Page:** 38

4 One-leg gym ball hamstring curl I **Sets:** 2
Reps: 10 each side **Page:** 73

5 T press-up I **Sets:** 2 **Reps:** 10 each side **Page:** 66

6 Gym ball dumb-bell triceps extension I **Sets:** 2
Reps: 10 each side **Page:** 55

7 Side plank star I **Sets:** 2 **Reps:** 10 each side **Page:** 30

Cluster workout

If you find that your training has plateaued, cluster workouts will inject new stimulus into your workouts. There are a number of ways of doing cluster workouts but essentially they all involve reducing the load so you can complete high reps with little rest. The result is that you lift a greater volume of weight during your session, which has a positive effect on muscle growth and calorie burn.

Designing your workout

One of the simplest ways to do a cluster workout is to do a normal workout until you get to the final two exercises. If you have done ten reps for each move, stick with a weight that you'd use to do ten reps for the final two moves if you were continuing your standard workout but only do five reps

of the penultimate exercise. Without resting, move on to the final exercise and do five reps. Go straight back to the penultimate exercise and alternate between the final two moves for five minutes, doing five reps of each without resting. Make sure you chose opposing or non-competing muscle groups such as legs and shoulders, otherwise you'll fatigue early.

Other ways of doing cluster workouts include doing single reps with your three-rep maximum with minimal rest between reps (ten seconds, say) or clusters of low-rep sets of one exercise with your ten-rep maximum with minimal rest between groups of reps. However you choose to arrange your workouts, this is an intense method so use it when you feel your progress has stalled.

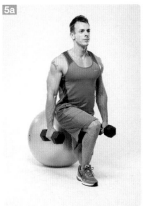

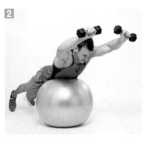

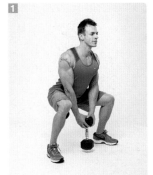

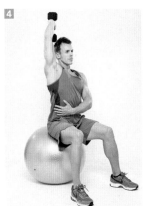

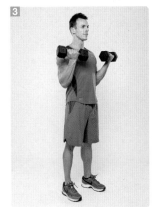

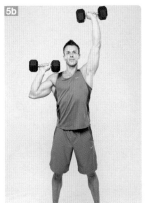

Cluster sample workout

1 Dumb-bell sumo squat | **Sets:** 3 **Reps:** 10 **Page:** 68

2 Gym ball lying Cuban press | **Sets:** 3 **Reps:** 10 **Page:** 79

3 Dumb-bell curl | **Sets:** 2 **Reps:** 10 each side **Page:** 52

4 Dumb-bell overhead triceps extension
Sets: 2 **Reps:** 10 each side **Page:** 55

5a Gym ball dumb-bell Bulgarian split squat
Cluster: 1 **Reps:** 5 each side **Page:** 71

5b Alternating dumb-bell shoulder press
Cluster: 1 **Reps:** 5 each side **Page:** 75

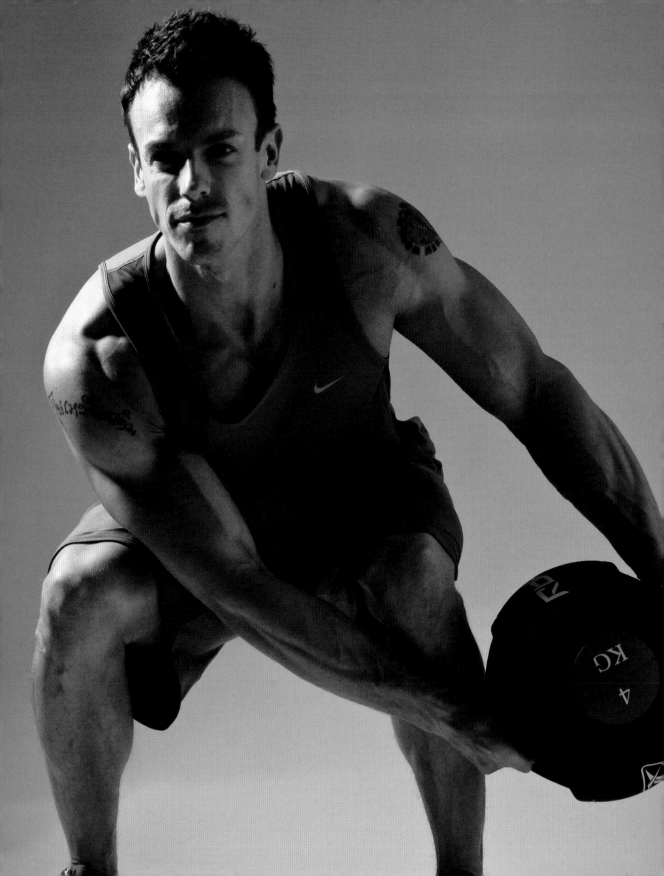

Extra kit
introduction

Explore new workout options by introducing three more bits of kit

Adding a pull-up bar, a medicine ball and a resistance band to your home gym will open up new areas of workout possibilities without taking over your spare room or using up all your spare cash. This chapter shows you the key moves you can do with these new bits of kit and how you can use them to create new workouts.

A pull-up bar lets you perform pull-ups and chin-ups, two of the most effective moves for building muscle.

A medicine ball lets you exercise dynamically to improve your co-ordination and balance and it can be thrown and caught without leaving dents in your floor or dislocations in your fingers. They can also be used to add resistance to bodyweight moves to make them sufficiently challenging to fatigue your muscles.

Resistance bands are different to other weights in your home gym stable because the resistance increases towards the top of the move, which challenges your muscles in a new way. They're also cheap and easy to store, which makes them a handy home workout tool.

Extra kit I Buyer's guide

Extra kit gear guide

Add a pull-up bar, medicine ball and resistance band to your home gym to expand your workout possibilities

Pull-up bar

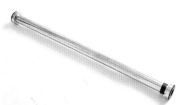

What it does

A pull-up bar will give you a great new muscle-building challenge. Performing pull-ups (where your palms face away from you) and chin-ups (where your palms face you) recruits a large number of muscles, making them a great muscle builder because they flood your body with growth hormones.

While you're hanging from the bar you're not in contact with the ground, which means that you have a bigger potential range of motion. You can also work your hard to reach lower abdominals, for an even development of your six-pack.

What to buy

The simplest bars can be adjusted to fit in a standard-size doorway. The downside is that you need to screw them into the frame to secure them in place. Some are designed to stay there permanently, others are more discreet and involve fixing two rubber circles to your frame, over which you slot an adjustable bar.

If tampering with woodwork isn't an option you can get bars that mount the doorframe without needing to be permanently secured. This option tends to be slightly more expensive, but obviously less instrusive.

Resistance band

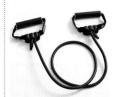

What it does

Resistance bands are ideal for home training because of their versatility. Think of them as a multi-gym without the weights – all you have to do is attach one end to something stable, such as a standing foot or a door, and start pulling or pushing, altering the length of band to vary the resistance.

They also work your muscles in a different way to training with freeweights. When using freeweights, resistance is greatest at the start of the move. It then reduces as you gather momentum towards the top of the move. With resistance bands, it's the other way round, so they challenge your muscles in a different way, which can result in new muscle growth.

What to buy

There are two main types of resistance band. The first comes without hand straps, is made of latex rubber and is also known as a stretchband. The other type is sometimes called a resistance tube and comes with handles at both ends of the band, which makes them easier to hold.

Resistance tubes come in different levels of resistance. You can either buy more than one and use different bands, or use the same band and adjust length of the part of the band you're stretching. The best resistance bands are ones that allow you to adjust the length of the band so you can create tension as required.

Medicine ball

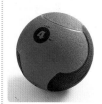

What it does

In the real world the body moves at high speed and creates momentum to make it easier to move objects. The faster you want to move something, the greater the speed and strength you need. This, essentially, is what we call power. Unfortunately, power is one of the most neglected aspects of training and few people possess the muscle synergy and tone to control their body's segments properly. That's where medicine balls come in. They allow you to add power to a workout in a natural way. And if you get bored of working out at home, you can use them outdoors.

What to buy

The weight of medicine ball you chose should depend on what exercises you're going to do with it. If you're relatively new to working out and you're only going to buy one ball, opt for 3kg. If you're more experienced go for 4kg or 5kg. Buying more than one ball will allow you to use the kit in exactly the way you want.

Leather balls look and feel nice but you can't use them outside. Balls with handles are good for certain exercises such as woodchops but are less good for throwing. Round rubber balls are nice to grip and easy to catch, and you won't feel guilty about slamming them on the floor.

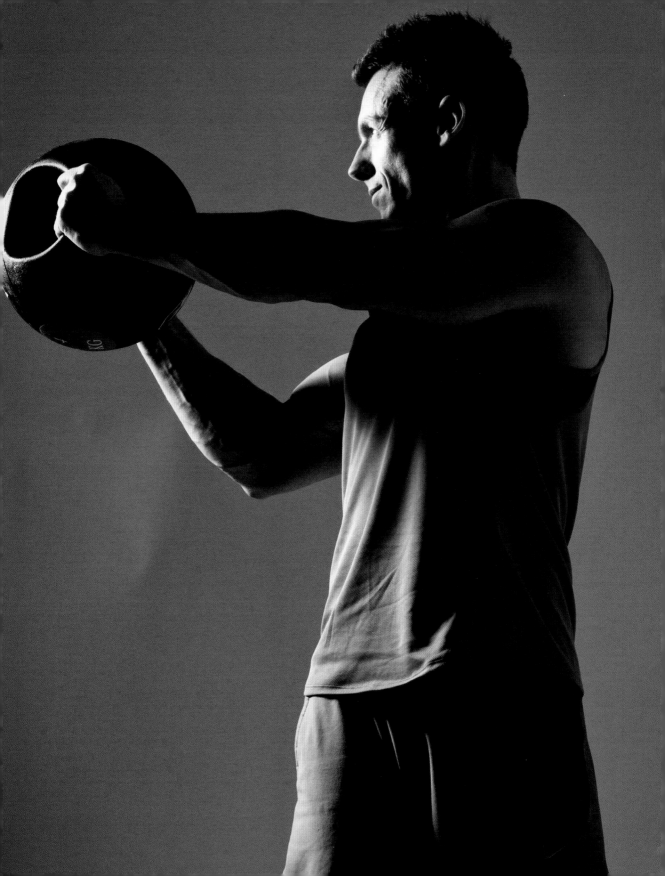

Extra kit **| Exercises**

01

Chin-up

Target:
biceps, lats
This challenging multi-joint move gives your biceps a real test and will also help to build a strong back.

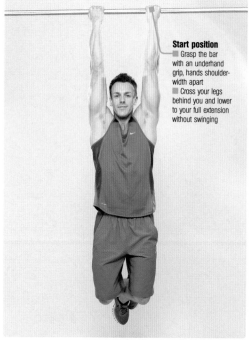

Start position
- Grasp the bar with an underhand grip, hands shoulder-width apart
- Cross your legs behind you and lower to your full extension without swinging

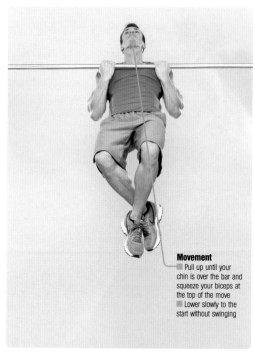

Movement
- Pull up until your chin is over the bar and squeeze your biceps at the top of the move
- Lower slowly to the start without swinging

02

Negative chin-up

Target:
biceps, lats
If you find chin-ups too difficult, try doing just the lowering phase by starting on a bench or getting a training partner to lift you to the up-phase of the move.

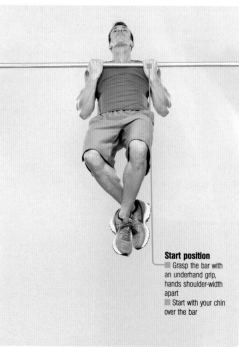

Start position
- Grasp the bar with an underhand grip, hands shoulder-width apart
- Start with your chin over the bar

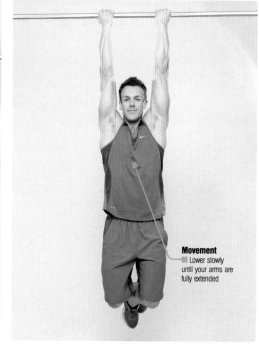

Movement
- Lower slowly until your arms are fully extended

Exercises | Extra kit

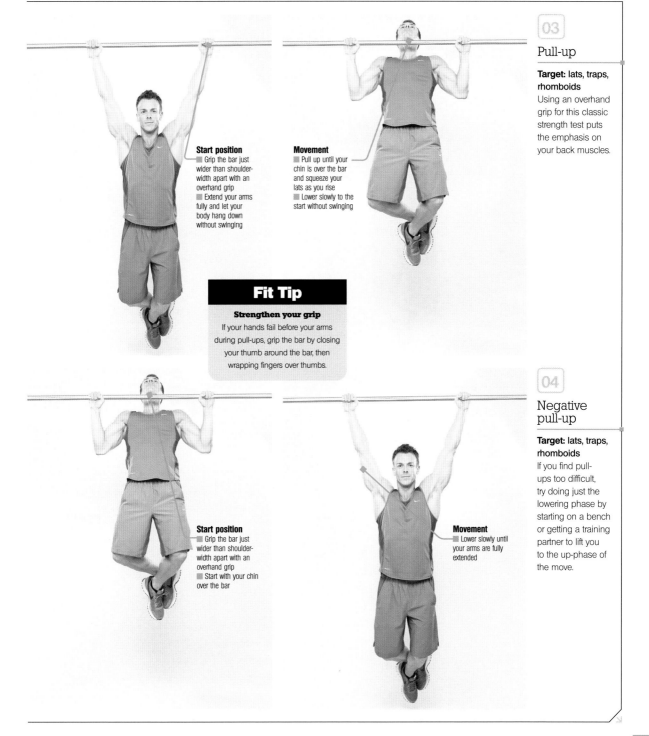

03

Pull-up

Target: lats, traps, rhomboids

Using an overhand grip for this classic strength test puts the emphasis on your back muscles.

Start position
■ Grip the bar just wider than shoulder-width apart with an overhand grip
■ Extend your arms fully and let your body hang down without swinging

Movement
■ Pull up until your chin is over the bar and squeeze your lats as you rise
■ Lower slowly to the start without swinging

Fit Tip

Strengthen your grip

If your hands fail before your arms during pull-ups, grip the bar by closing your thumb around the bar, then wrapping fingers over thumbs.

04

Negative pull-up

Target: lats, traps, rhomboids

If you find pull-ups too difficult, try doing just the lowering phase by starting on a bench or getting a training partner to lift you to the up-phase of the move.

Start position
■ Grip the bar just wider than shoulder-width apart with an overhand grip
■ Start with your chin over the bar

Movement
■ Lower slowly until your arms are fully extended

Extra kit **I** Exercises

05

Wide-grip pull-up

Target: lats, traps, rhomboids
Widening your grip makes the move harder and puts more of an emphasis on your lats.

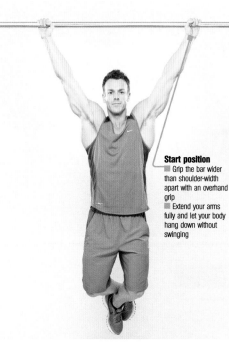

Start position
- Grip the bar wider than shoulder-width apart with an overhand grip
- Extend your arms fully and let your body hang down without swinging

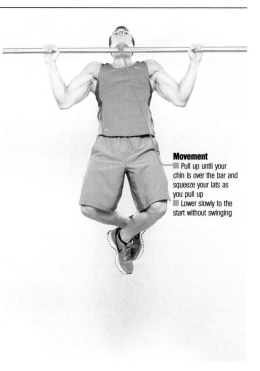

Movement
- Pull up until your chin is over the bar and squeeze your lats as you pull up
- Lower slowly to the start without swinging

06

Hanging knee raise

Target: lower abdominals
Work the often-neglected lower abdominals to help carve a six-pack.

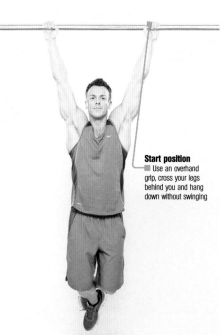

Start position
- Use an overhand grip, cross your legs behind you and hang down without swinging

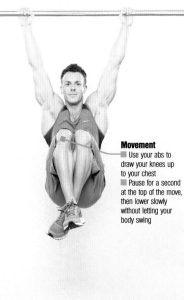

Movement
- Use your abs to draw your knees up to your chest
- Pause for a second at the top of the move, then lower slowly without letting your body swing

Exercises I Extra kit

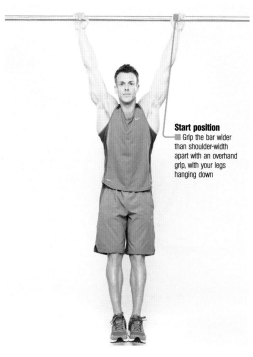

Start position
- Grip the bar wider than shoulder-width apart with an overhand grip, with your legs hanging down

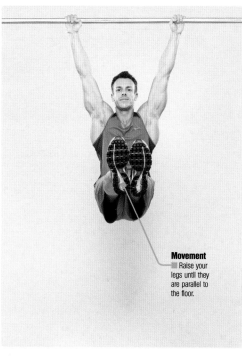

Movement
- Raise your legs until they are parallel to the floor.

07

Hanging leg raise

Target: lower abdominals
Keeping your legs straight as you raise them up is tougher than the knee raise but is great for strengthening your lower abs.

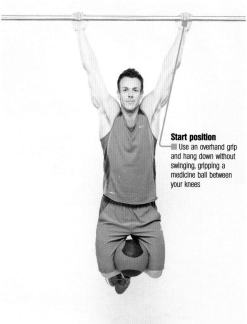

Start position
- Use an overhand grip and hang down without swinging, gripping a medicine ball between your knees

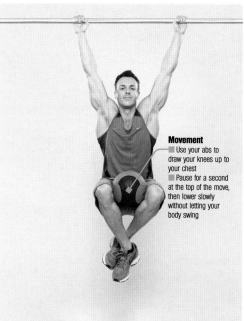

Movement
- Use your abs to draw your knees up to your chest
- Pause for a second at the top of the move, then lower slowly without letting your body swing

08

Medicine ball knee raise

Target: lower abdominals
Using a medicine ball makes knee raises more challenging, allowing you to fatigue at your desired rep range once you're good at standard knee raises.

Extra kit | Exercises

09

Twisting knee raise

Target: lower abs, obliques
Bring your side abs into play for a more complete core workout by twisting as you raise your knees.

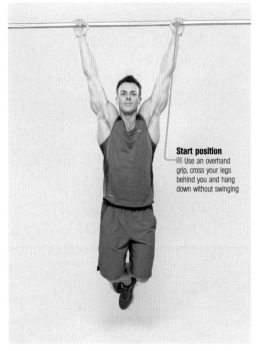

Start position
- Use an overhand grip, cross your legs behind you and hang down without swinging

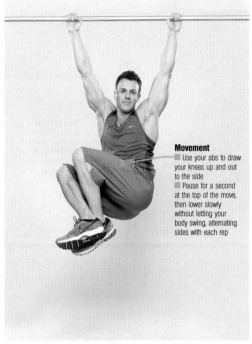

Movement
- Use your abs to draw your knees up and out to the side
- Pause for a second at the top of the move, then lower slowly without letting your body swing, alternating sides with each rep

10

Climbers chin-ups

Target: lats, traps, rhomboids
You don't have to be a climber to get the benefits of this move, which increases upper-body strength and shoulder-joint stabilisation.

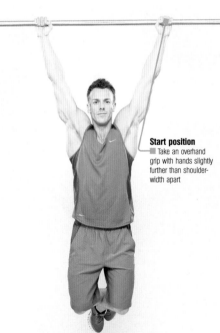

Start position
- Take an overhand grip with hands slightly further than shoulder-width apart

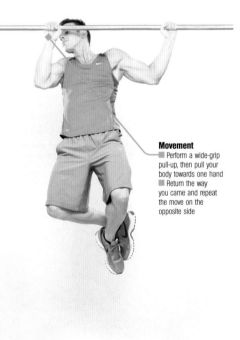

Movement
- Perform a wide-grip pull-up, then pull your body towards one hand
- Return the way you came and repeat the move on the opposite side

Exercises | Extra kit

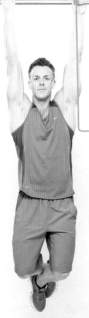

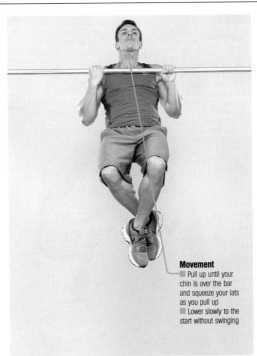

11

Mixed-grip pull-up

Target: lats, traps, rhomboids, biceps, core
Taking a mixed grip makes your body control the rotational force for a stronger core.

Start position
- Grab a pull-up bar with a mixed grip – one palm facing you, the other facing away from you
- Extend your arms fully and let your body hang down without swinging

Movement
- Pull up until your chin is over the bar and squeeze your lats as you pull up
- Lower slowly to the start without swinging

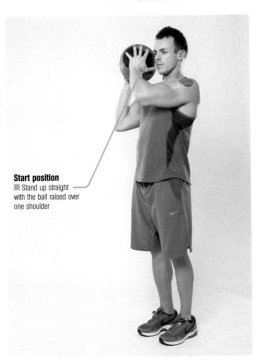

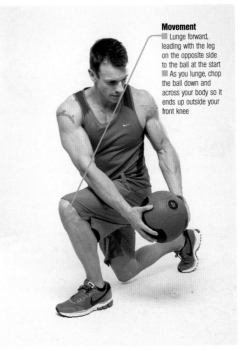

12

Medicine ball lunge chop

Target: whole body
This move is a great test of balance and coordination. Holding the lunge position makes your core work overtime as it tries to stabilise your hips and torso.

Movement
- Lunge forward, leading with the leg on the opposite side to the ball at the start
- As you lunge, chop the ball down and across your body so it ends up outside your front knee

Start position
- Stand up straight with the ball raised over one shoulder

Extra kit I Exercises

13

Medicine ball woodchop

Target: whole body

This move recruits the whole body to lift the ball but does it all through the core so that the muscles in your midriff put in a massive effort.

Start position
■ Start with your back flat, your core engaged and your feet shoulder-width apart
■ Your knees should be in line with your feet with your thighs almost parallel to the floor
■ Hold a medicine ball in both hands on the outside of your thigh

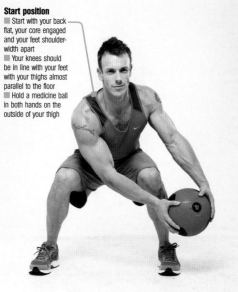

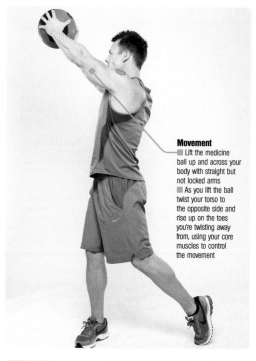

Movement
■ Lift the medicine ball up and across your body with straight but not locked arms
■ As you lift the ball twist your torso to the opposite side and rise up on the toes you're twisting away from, using your core muscles to control the movement

14

Medicine ball reverse crunch

Target: lower abdominals

Adding extra weight to a reverse crunch will allow you to build extra muscle.

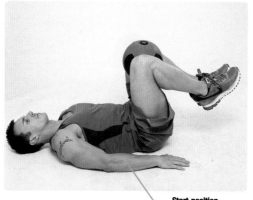

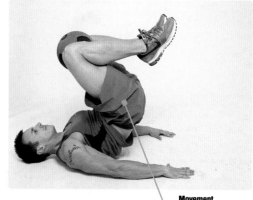

Start position
■ Lie with your head and back on the floor and your arms out by your sides for support
■ Your knees should be bent so that your thighs are vertical
■ Grip a medicine ball between your legs

Movement
■ Contract your abs to lift your hips off the floor
■ Pause at the top of the move then lower slowly back to the start

Exercises | Extra kit

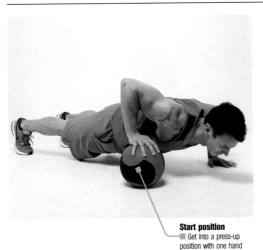

Start position
- Get into a press-up position with one hand on the medicine ball underneath your shoulder

Movement
- Push up and pass the ball across to your other hand
- Pass the ball back and forth with each press-up

15

Medicine ball passing press-up

Target: chest, triceps, core
Using a medicine ball increases the push and forces you to stabilise your shoulder joint.

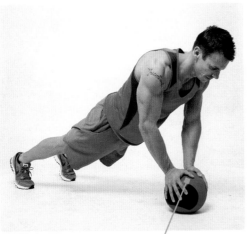

Start position
- Get into a press-up position with both hands on top of the ball

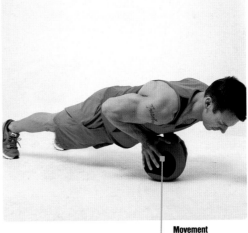

Movement
- Lower down then press up, using your core muscles to prevent the ball from moving

16

Medicine ball close grip press-up

Target: chest, triceps, core
Positioning both hands on top of the medicine ball ramps up the demand placed on your core and shoulders.

Extra kit **I** Exercises

17

Medicine ball side throwdowns

Target: obliques
The throwing action works your side abs plyometrically, developing your fast-twitch muscles and increasing your power production.

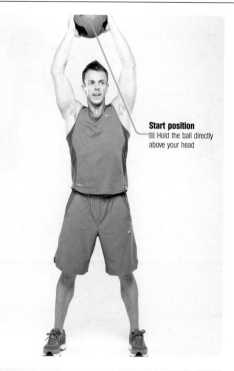

Start position
■ Hold the ball directly above your head

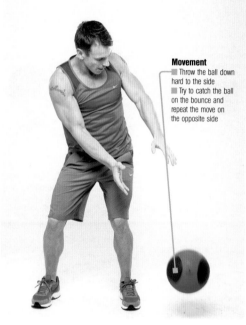

Movement
■ Throw the ball down hard to the side
■ Try to catch the ball on the bounce and repeat the move on the opposite side

18

Medicine ball leg drop

Target: lower abs, hips, adductors
Increase the resistance of a standard leg drop by placing a medicine ball between your feet.

Start position
■ Lie on your back with your head and shoulders on the floor and your arms flat on the floor for balance
■ Grip a medicine ball between your feet with your legs up in the air

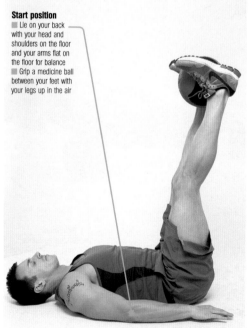

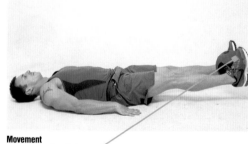

Movement
■ Lower the ball as slowly as you can under control
■ Stop before your heels touch the floor and return to the start

Fit Tip

Target your lower abs
The lower section of the abs is the one that's most difficult to hit. To make sure you get a six-pack rather than just a four pack, do leg drops with a medicine ball.

Exercises **|** Extra kit

Start position
■ Stand with your feet shoulder-width apart, your knees bent slightly, and lean forwards from the hips, not the waist
■ Keeping your back straight and your shoulder blades retracted, hold a medicine ball in both hands with your arms hanging straight down

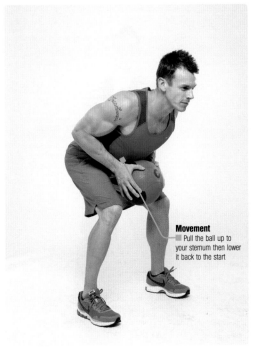

Movement
■ Pull the ball up to your sternum then lower it back to the start

19

Medicine ball bent-over row

Target: lats, traps, rhomboids
Work your back with the medicine ball variation of the classic big muscle-building move.

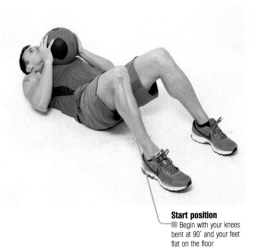

Start position
■ Begin with your knees bent at 90˚ and your feet flat on the floor
■ Hold the medicine ball on your chest with your head slightly off the floor

Movement
■ Contract your abs to lift your shoulders off the floor without straining at the neck
■ Keep your lower back in contact with the floor and curl your chest towards your knees
■ Pause at the top of the move to squeeze your abs and lower slowly to the start

20

Medicine ball crunch

Target: abdominals
Using a medicine ball to perform a crunch makes the move harder so you can fatigue your muscles without doing an excessively high number of repetitions.

Extra kit **|** Exercises

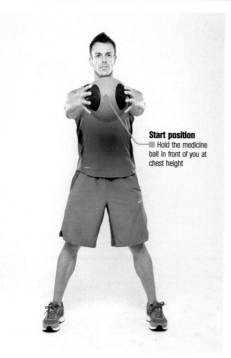

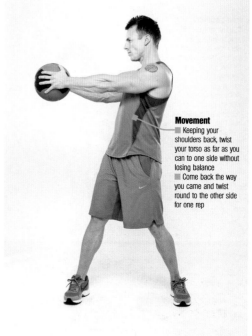

21

Medicine ball tornado chop

Target: obliques
This dynamic move targets your side abs and will get your heart rate up for a fat-burning effect.

Start position
■ Hold the medicine ball in front of you at chest height

Movement
■ Keeping your shoulders back, twist your torso as far as you can to one side without losing balance
■ Come back the way you came and twist round to the other side for one rep

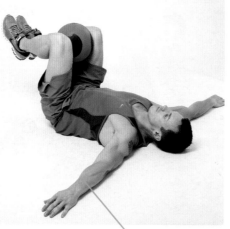

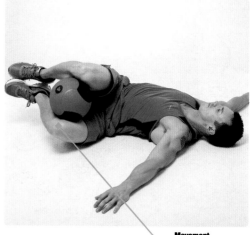

22

Medicine ball Russian twist

Target: lower abs, obliques
This move challenges two areas of your mid-section that are easily neglected – the lower abs and obliques.

Start position
■ Lie with your back, head and shoulders on the floor with your arms out to the sides for balance
■ Hold a medicine ball between your knees with your knees bent at 90° and your thighs vertical

Movement
■ Lower your legs under control to one side without your shoulders leaving the floor
■ Stop before your legs touch the floor and return to the start the way you came before lowering to the other side

Exercises | Extra kit

Start position
■ Squat with the ball in both hands between your legs

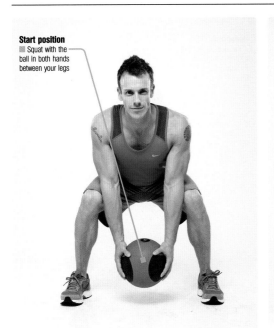

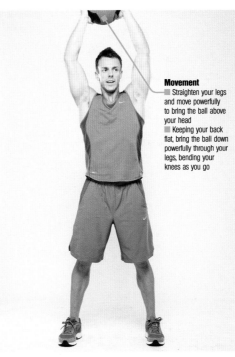

Movement
■ Straighten your legs and move powerfully to bring the ball above your head
■ Keeping your back flat, bring the ball down powerfully through your legs, bending your knees as you go

23

Medicine ball sledge-hammer

Target: whole body
This dynamic move will get muscle firing all over your body and is great for stabilising your lower back.

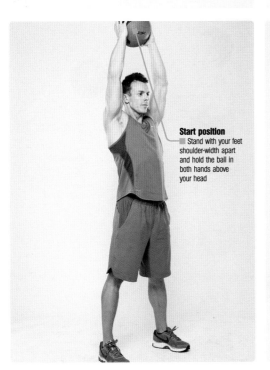

Start position
■ Stand with your feet shoulder-width apart and hold the ball in both hands above your head

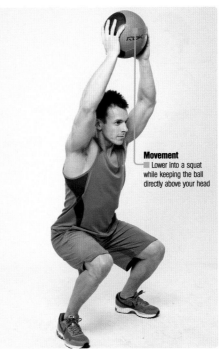

Movement
■ Lower into a squat while keeping the ball directly above your head

24

Medicine ball overhead squat

Target: quads, hamstrings, glutes
Use a medicine ball to test your shoulder stability before moving on to doing the exercise with a barbell.

Extra kit **|** Exercises

25

Medicine ball walking lunge

Target: whole body

Develop your balance and coordination while working a range of muscle groups with this functional move.

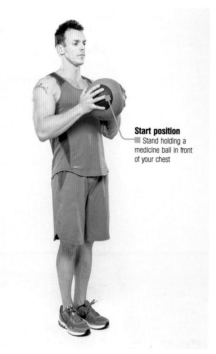

Start position
■ Stand holding a medicine ball in front of your chest

Movement
■ Step forward into a lunge and, as you do so, push the medicine ball out in front of you
■ Bring your back leg through to stand up straight and pull the ball back into your chest
■ Lunge forward with the opposite leg to repeat the move

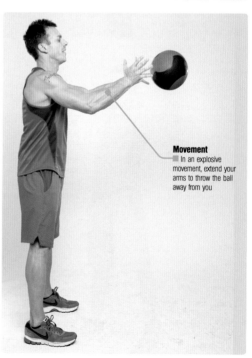

26

Medicine ball wall throw

Target: chest, triceps

Throwing the ball at a wall or at a partner makes it a plyometric move, which will develop your fast-twitch muscle fibres and increase your explosive force production.

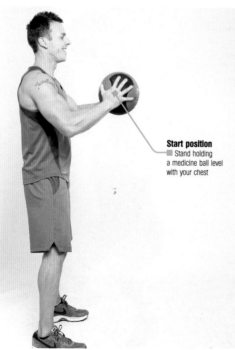

Start position
■ Stand holding a medicine ball level with your chest

Movement
■ In an explosive movement, extend your arms to throw the ball away from you

Exercises **|** Extra kit

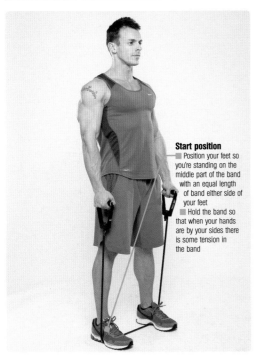

Start position
- Position your feet so you're standing on the middle part of the band with an equal length of band either side of your feet
- Hold the band so that when your hands are by your sides there is some tension in the band

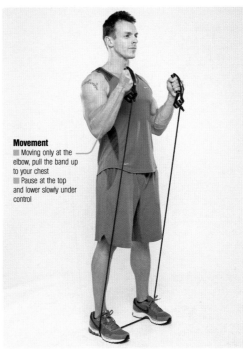

Movement
- Moving only at the elbow, pull the band up to your chest
- Pause at the top and lower slowly under control

27

Hammer curl

Target: biceps
Doing a hammer curl as opposed to a straight biceps curl takes the emphasis away from your biceps brachii and poses more of a challenge to your forearms.

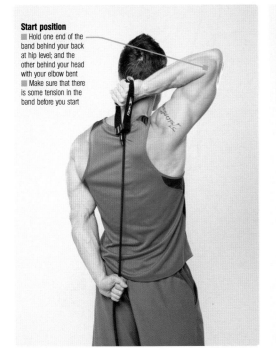

Start position
- Hold one end of the band behind your back at hip level; and the other behind your head with your elbow bent
- Make sure that there is some tension in the band before you start

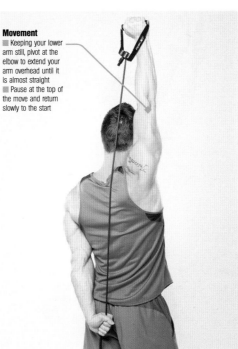

Movement
- Keeping your lower arm still, pivot at the elbow to extend your arm overhead until it is almost straight
- Pause at the top of the move and return slowly to the start

28

Triceps extension

Target: triceps
Isolate the backs of your arms with this single joint move.

Extra kit I Exercises

29
One-arm shoulder press

Target: shoulders
Doing this as a one-arm move brings your core into play as it works to keep your torso stable.

Start position
■ Anchor one end of the band under one foot and grasp the handle with the hand on the same side, palm facing away from you at shoulder height

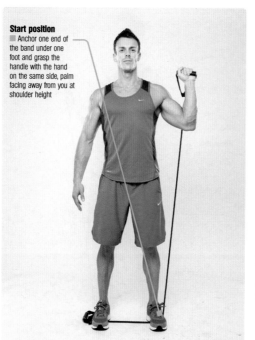

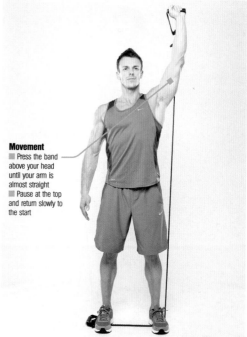

Movement
■ Press the band above your head until your arm is almost straight
■ Pause at the top and return slowly to the start

30
Lat pull-down

Target: lats, biceps
Hook the band over the top of a door to build a stronger back.

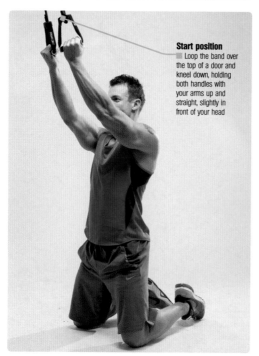

Start position
■ Loop the band over the top of a door and kneel down, holding both handles with your arms up and straight, slightly in front of your head

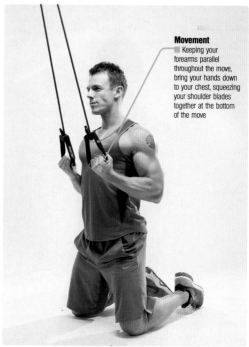

Movement
■ Keeping your forearms parallel throughout the move, bring your hands down to your chest, squeezing your shoulder blades together at the bottom of the move

Exercises I Extra kit

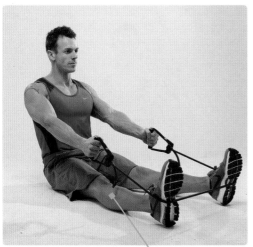

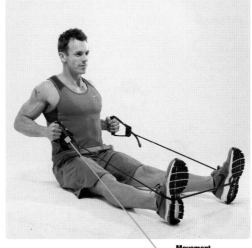

31

Seated row

Target: traps, lats, rhomboids
Work your back muscles with this simple but effective move.

Start position
- Sit with your legs straight and make sure that there is tension in the band when you loop it round the soles of your feet and your arms are out in front of you

Movement
- Pull the band back until your hands are level with your chest
- Squeeze your shoulder blades together at the top of the move and return slowly to the start

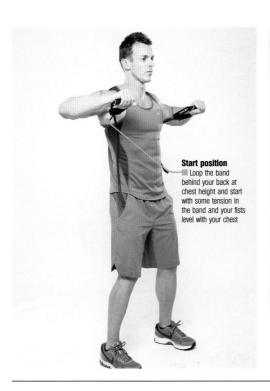

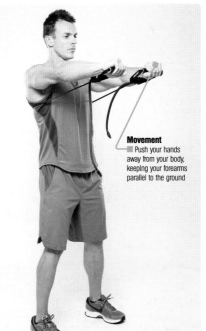

32

Standing chest press

Target: chest
Adapt this classic move by looping the band around your back to develop your chest.

Start position
- Loop the band behind your back at chest height and start with some tension in the band and your fists level with your chest

Movement
- Push your hands away from your body, keeping your forearms parallel to the ground

Extra kit **|** Exercises

Squats

Target: quads, glutes, hamstrings
Using a resistance band to do squats increases the resistance as you stand up, working your muscles in a different way to a pair of dumb-bells or a barbell.

Start position
■ Stand on the band and hold it so that there's tension in the band when you're in the down position of a squat

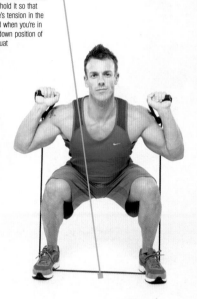

Movement
■ Keeping your back straight, push up through your heels to a standing position then lower slowly back to the start

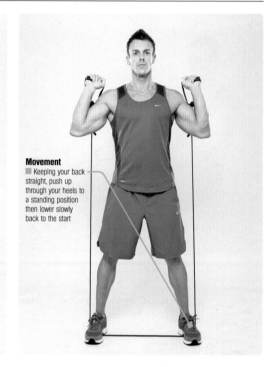

Leg curl

Target: hamstrings
Work the backs of your legs to balance the quad-dominant work you do when performing squats.

Start position
■ Secure the handle of one end of the band around one of your feet and stand on the band with your other foot so that there's tension on the band when the toes on the working leg are level with the heel of the standing leg
■ Keep the knee of your working leg tucked into the other knee

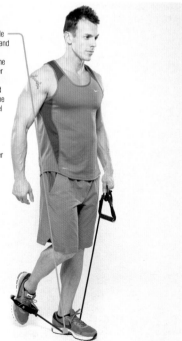

Movement
■ Slowly raise your heel behind you for the full range of movement, keeping your toes pointing down
■ Control the movement back to the start and swap legs each set

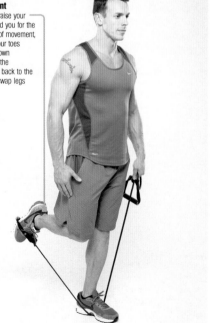

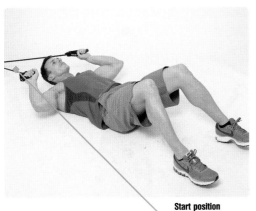

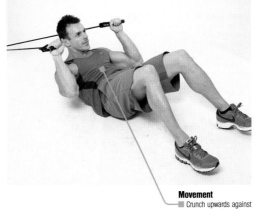

35

Crunch

Target:
abdominals
The resistance
band increases
the difficulty of the
move so you can
work your abs even
harder.

Start position
- Loop the band around a solid structure such as a table leg
- Lie on the floor with your back to the table and hold the band by the handles so that there's tension in it before you start the crunch

Movement
- Crunch upwards against the resistance of the band, pause and lower yourself under control, avoiding touching your shoulders to the floor between reps

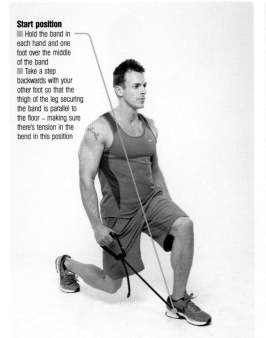

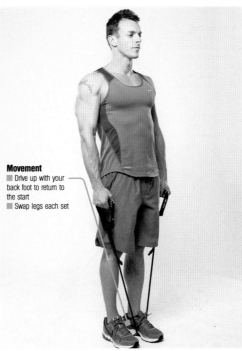

36

Lunge

**Target: glutes,
quads, hamstrings**
Work your entire
lower body with
this dynamic move
that tests your
coordination.

Start position
- Hold the band in each hand and one foot over the middle of the band
- Take a step backwards with your other foot so that the thigh of the leg securing the band is parallel to the floor – making sure there's tension in the bend in this position

Movement
- Drive up with your back foot to return to the start
- Swap legs each set

Extra kit I **Exercises**

37

Lateral raise

Target: deltoids
This move will strengthen your shoulders and make them look broader.

Start position
■ Stand with one foot slightly in front of the other and the band beneath it
■ Hold one end of the band in each hand with your arms down by your sides

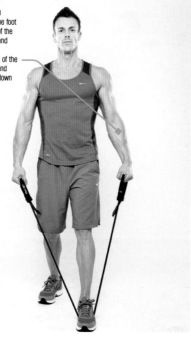

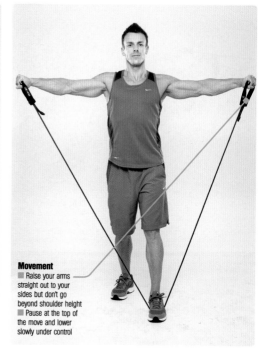

Movement
■ Raise your arms straight out to your sides but don't go beyond shoulder height
■ Pause at the top of the move and lower slowly under control

38

Woodchop

Target: whole body
Use this dynamic movement to build a strong core and improve your upper-to-lower body force transfer.

Start position
■ Stand on the band with your feet slightly wider than shoulder-width apart and your knees slightly bent.
■ Hold the handles in both hands

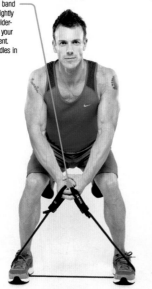

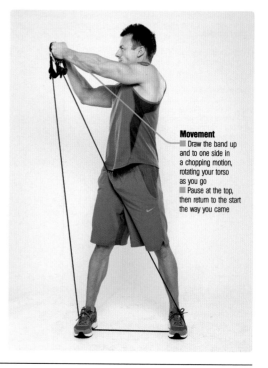

Movement
■ Draw the band up and to one side in a chopping motion, rotating your torso as you go
■ Pause at the top, then return to the start the way you came

Exercises | Extra kit

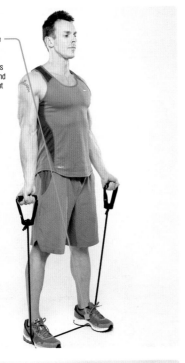

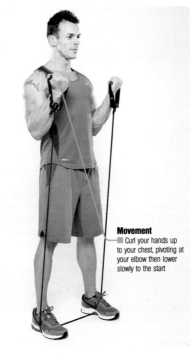

Start position
- Stand on top of the band with your feet shoulder-width apart
- Start with your arms down by your sides and your palms facing front with some tension in the band

Movement
- Curl your hands up to your chest, pivoting at your elbow then lower slowly to the start

39

Biceps curl

Target: biceps
Using a resistance band will work your muscles in a different way to using dumb-bells, giving you new muscle growth for this classic move.

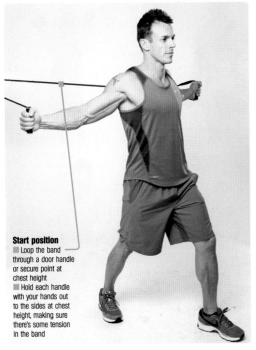

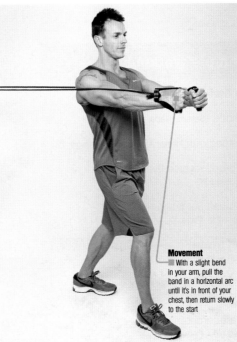

Start position
- Loop the band through a door handle or secure point at chest height
- Hold each handle with your hands out to the sides at chest height, making sure there's some tension in the band

Movement
- With a slight bend in your arm, pull the band in a horizontal arc until it's in front of your chest, then return slowly to the start

40

Chest flye

Target: chest
This move takes the focus away from your arm muscles and concentrates it on your chest.

Extra kit **I** Workouts

Full-body workout

Incorporating your new bits of kit into your full-body workouts will increase your workout options. That, in turn, will make you less likely to plateau and more likely to continue to build muscle.

Even with a broader range of kit involved, full-body workouts are still an efficient way of working out because they allow you to work a large range of muscle fibres in a relatively short space of time. You may find it difficult to fully exhaust your muscle fibres during full-body workouts but you can combine them with body focus workouts (an example of which is opposite).

Designing your workouts

The important thing to remember when designing full-body workouts is that they need to be balanced. So, for every pushing motion you should do a pulling one, and you should spend as much time on your upper body as you do on your lower. Stick to compound moves (the ones that work several muscle groups at once) because these will give you maximum muscle development.

Leave any abs moves to the end of your workout because you don't want them to be fatigued when you perform big moves such as pull-ups.

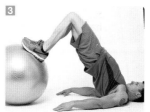
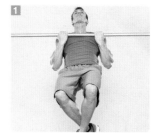
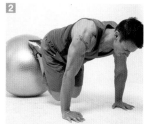
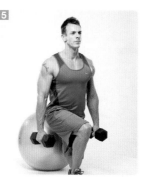
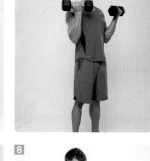
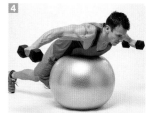
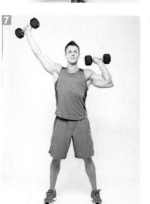
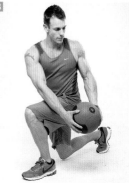

Full-body sample workout

1 Pull-up **I Sets: 3 Reps: 8 Page: 107**

2 Gym ball jackknife **I Sets: 3 Reps: 10-12 Page: 59**

3 Gym ball hamstring curl **I Sets: 3 Reps: 10-12 Page: 72**

4 Gym ball dumb-bell reverse flye
Sets: 3 Reps: 10-12 Page: 63

5 Gym ball dumb-bell Bulgarian split squat
Sets: 2 Reps: 10 each side Page: 71

6 Hammer curl with twist
Sets: 2 Reps: 10 each side Page: 54

7 Alternating wide shoulder press
Sets: 2 Reps: 10 each side Page: 76

8 Medicine ball lunge chop
Sets: 2 Reps: 10 each side Page: 111

Body focus workout

By focusing on one body part you can completely fatigue the target muscle. You should then let that body part recover for a week while you train different muscles. It's a good way of being specific about how you put on muscle but the downside is that doing lots of single-joint exercises won't produce as big a growth hormone release as doing big compound moves in a full-body workout. You also need to be prepared to exercise frequently if you want to work every major muscle group once a week.

Designing your workouts

It's important that you get your session structure right for body focus workouts. If you get it wrong, you increase your chances of overtraining or risking injury.

Start by doing light exercises that will warm up your joint before moving on to do the bigger muscle-building moves. You must then make sure you have fully fatigued the muscle by doing a single-joint move. Vary the exercises and angles you use to work that body part so that you get good and well balanced muscle growth.

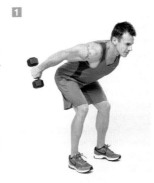

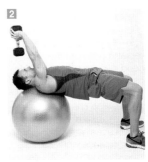

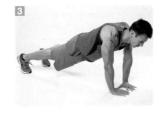

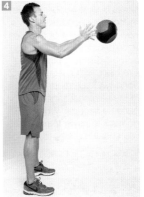

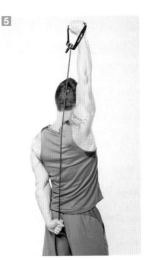

Body focus sample workout: triceps

1 Two-arm dumb-bell kickback
Sets: 2 **Reps:** 10 **Page:** 56

2 Gym ball lying triceps extension
Sets: 2 **Reps:** 10 **Page:** 55

3 Diamond press-up I **Sets:** 2 **Reps:** 10 **Page:** 35

4 Medicine ball wall throw I **Sets:** 2 **Reps:** 10 **Page:** 118

5 Resistance band triceps extension
Sets: 2 **Reps:** 8 each side **Page:** 119

Extra kit I **Workouts**

Resistance band workout

The big appeal of resistance bands is that they are portable and versatile. They are therefore good if you're going travelling but don't want to take a break from exercising.

They also challenge your muscles in a different way to conventional weights because the resistance increases towards the top of a move. This is the exact opposite to conventional weights, which become easier to lift at the top of the move as momentum kicks in. The different type of stress is useful because you're muscles respond best to new stimulus. If your muscles have become used to lifting dumb-bells, doing the same exercises with a resistance band will force them to adapt to the new challenge to become stronger. When you go back to using dumb-bells, you should be able to lift more.

Designing your workouts

You can use a resistance band to do virtually all the workout options outlined in this book. If you want to do a superset workout, for example, simply arrange your exercises and rest periods in the same way you'd construct the workout if you were using other items of kit.

Some workouts, such as drop sets or back-off sets, aren't ideally suited to resistance bands because it's best to be precise about how much weight you're lifting. You can, however, make any exercise easier or harder depending on the length and resistance of the band, so it is still possible to use those techniques.

The workout sample on this page is for a full-body workout but you can design your resistance band routine to meet your workout goals.

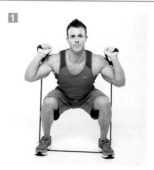

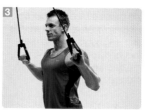

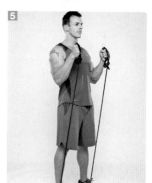

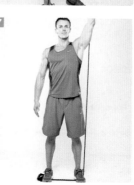

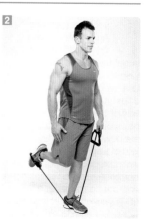

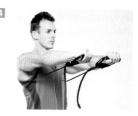

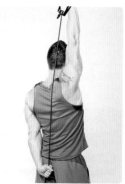

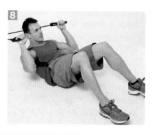

Resistance band sample workout

1 Squat I **Sets:** 3 **Reps:** 10-12 **Page:** 122

2 Leg curl I **Sets:** 2 **Reps:** 10 each side **Page:** 122

3 Lat pull-down I **Sets:** 3 **Reps:** 10-12 **Page:** 120

4 Chest press I **Sets:** 3 **Reps:** 10-12 **Page:** 121

5 Hammer curl I **Sets:** 2 **Reps:** 10 each side **Page:** 119

6 Triceps extension I **Sets:** 2 **Reps:** 10 each side **Page:** 119

7 Shoulder press I **Sets:** 2 **Reps:** 10 each side **Page:** 120

8 Crunch I **Sets:** 3 **Reps:** 10-12 **Page:** 123

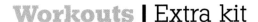
Workouts | Extra kit

Medicine ball workout

Medicine balls are an underrated item of home gym kit. They're surprisingly versatile and, unlike a set of dumb-bells, can be thrown around.

Because they're easy to hold, medicine balls are great for doing dynamic moves such as walking lunges, which develop your balance and proprioception – the ability of your body to sense and control its movement. They can also introduce an added element of instability to standard moves such as press-ups, which will strengthen the stabilising muscles in your joints and prepare you for big barbell lifts.

If bodyweight exercises such as crunches become too easy, you can use a medicine ball to increase the resistance and fatigue your muscles within a hypertrophy rep range.

Designing your workouts

You can use a medicine ball to do several of the workout options throughout this book. It is, however, probably best suited to either full-body workouts (because you can target every major group), core-stability workouts (because medicine balls are great at introducing instability and developing balance) and for circuit workouts (because you can use them for every exercise and they won't fatigue your muscles too quickly).

The sample workout on this page is a full-body session but if you want to use a medicine ball to do a different kind of workout, simply arrange your exercises and rest periods in the same way you'd construct the workout if you were using other items of kit.

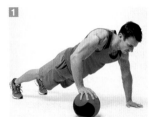

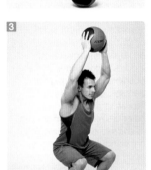

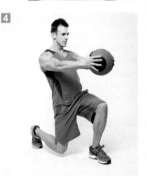

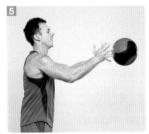

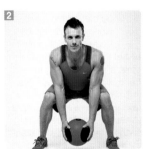

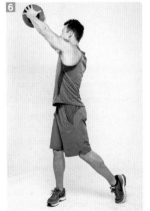

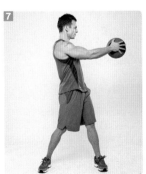

Medicine ball sample workout

1 Passing medicine ball press-up
Sets: 2 **Reps:** 10 each side **Page:** 113

2 Medicine ball sledgehammer
Sets: 3 **Reps:** 12 **Page:** 117

3 Medicine ball overhead squat
Sets: 3 **Reps:** 12 **Page:** 117

4 Medicine ball walking lunge
Sets: 2 **Reps:** 10 each side **Page:** 118

5 Medicine ball wall throw | **Sets:** 1 **Time:** 1 minute **Page:** 118

6 Medicine ball woodchop
Sets: 2 **Reps:** 10 each side **Page:** 112

7 Medicine ball tornado chop | **Sets:** 3 **Reps:** 12 **Page:** 116

Extra kit | Workouts

Circuit training workout

You can create a circuit workout using either bodyweight or minimal kit but introducing a new item of kit, such as a resistance band, will test your muscles in a different way. This will give you a new training effect, although circuits are still most suitable for people who want to lose fat rather than increase muscle size.

The key theory remains the same whatever kit you use. Doing different exercises back to back with no rest keeps your effort level high and forces your heart to pump blood to different parts of your body, giving you both a cardiovascular and a muscle-building benefit.

Designing your workouts

For circuits to be at their most effective, you need to move from one exercise to the next as swiftly as possible, which is why it's best to do all the moves in the workout with one item of kit.

Pick a group of exercises that target as many different muscle groups as possible and alternate between upper and lower body moves to make your heart work harder without experiencing excessive muscle fatigue. Include a good mix of pushing, pulling, lunging, bending and rotational moves to give your workout balance. You should also try to complete the reps quickly but without compromising good form. Once you have completed the circuit, rest for three minutes, then do it all again. The fitter you become, the more circuits you'll be able to complete.

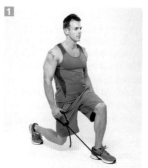
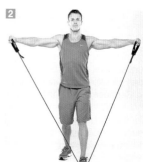
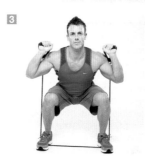
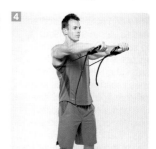
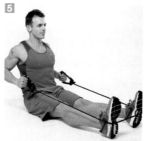
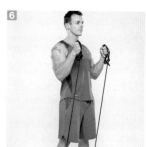
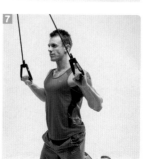
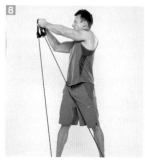

Resistance band circuit training sample workout

1 Lunge | **Sets:** 1 **Reps:** 10 each side **Page:** 123

2 Lateral raise | **Sets:** 1 **Reps:** 10 **Page:** 124

3 Squat | **Sets:** 1 **Reps:** 10 **Page:** 122

4 Chest press | **Sets:** 1 **Reps:** 10 **Page:** 121

5 Seated row | **Sets:** 1 **Reps:** 10 **Page:** 121

6 Hammer curl | **Sets:** 1 **Reps:** 10 each side **Page:** 119

7 Lat pull-down | **Sets:** 1 **Reps:** 10 **Page:** 120

8 Woodchop | **Sets:** 1 **Reps:** 10 each side **Page:** 124

Core stability workout

Good core stability is essential if you want to lift heavy weights, be better at sport and stay injury free. Your core muscles are the ones around your midriff, including your abdominals and lower back, and their function is to provide a link between your upper and lower body. They're particularly important during whole-body moves, which need a strong core to transfer power from upper to lower body. They're also called upon to stabilise your spine during dynamic and sporty movements.

A weak core will inhibit your ability to lift heavy weights in whole-body moves because you won't be able to transfer force from your lower to upper body. You may also suffer from lower-back and postural problems.

Designing your workouts

To get a strong and stable midsection you need to attack your core from different angles and target the muscles at the sides and back of your midriff. Start with moves that place the greatest weight on your core, such as compound lifts, and end with bodyweight exercises that won't risk injuring your tired muscles. Because this workout focuses on stability, you should complete a relatively high number of reps per set.

Using extra items of kit such as a resistance band will have a positive effect on your core strength because they allow you to challenge your muscles in a new way. A knee raise on a pull-up bar, for example, works your lower abdominals, which are harder to target than your upper abs.

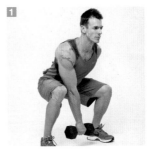

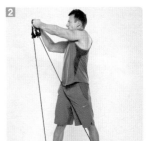

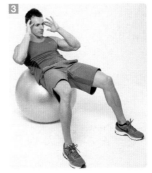

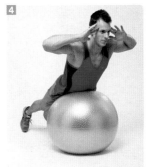

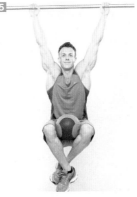

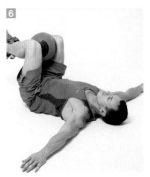

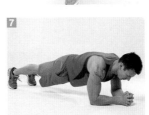

Core stability sample workout

1 Dumb-bell snatch I **Sets: 2 Reps:** 10-12 **Page:** 81

2 Resistance band woodchop
Sets: 2 Reps: 10-12 each arm **Page:** 124

3 Gym ball crunch I **Sets: 2 Reps:** 15 **Page:** 57

4 Gym ball back extension I **Sets: 2 Reps:** 15 **Page:** 62

5 Medicine ball knee raise I **Sets: 2 Reps:** 15 **Page:** 109

6 Medicine ball Russian twist
Sets: 2 Reps: 15 each side **Page:** 116

7 Plank I **Sets: 1 Time:** hold as long as possible **Page:** 29

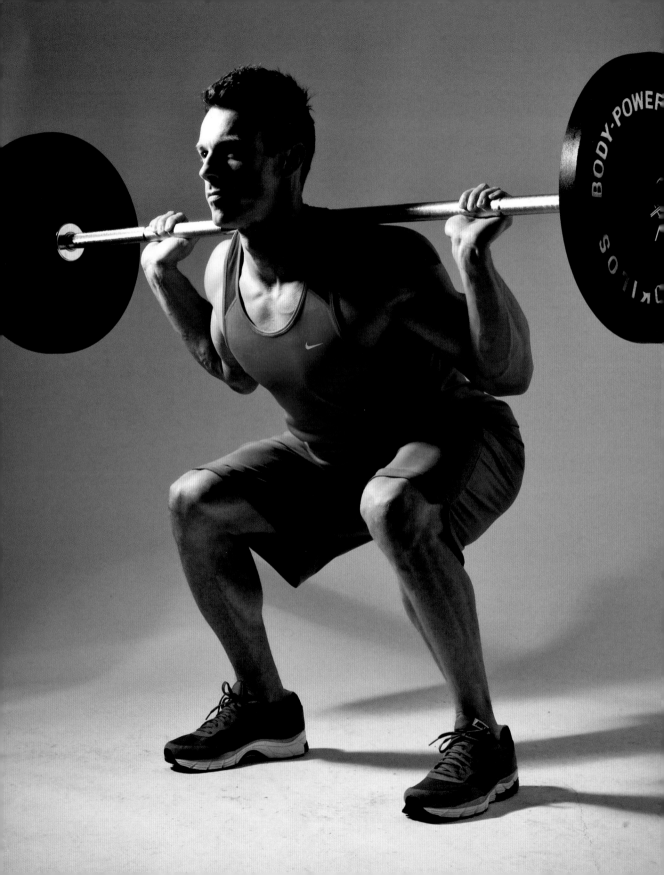

Barbell & bench
introduction

Lift heavy weights and pack on muscle with a barbell and bench

If you're really serious about getting bigger and stronger, a good barbell and bench will give you maximum muscle growth. This chapter will give you an arsenal of big muscle moves and show you how to use your bench and bar – as well as how to combine them with the other pieces of kit in the book – to achieve the body you want.

Once you get used to exercising with dumb-bells, you may find that you need to graduate to lifting something heavier for big compound moves such as squats and deadlifts. A barbell will let you load up the weights, which in turn will have a positive effect on the size and strength of your muscles. Some big barbell lifts, such as a bench press, require a bench because you need a solid base upon which to perform the move.

Barbell & bench I Buyer's guide

Barbell and bench gear guide

Get ready to start lifting heavy by using a barbell and bench

Bench

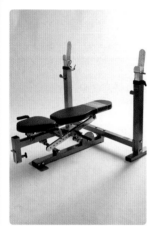

What it does

There's a reason why you don't see people doing heavy barbell chest presses on a gym ball. A bench offers you a stable platform for big lifts so you can use heavy weights without worrying about losing control.

There are two main types of bench: utility benches, which are just a platform, and bench press benches, which have a barbell cradle to hold a barbell above where your head rests on a bench. If you want to lift heavy weights

without a spotter, go for a bench press option.

What to look for

The bench needs to be stable when you're lying on it and, more importantly, lifting a heavy weight. If it creaks and strains, you'll be more worried about ending up in a heap of metal than you are about using perfect form.

A bench with a good incline and decline range will increase the range of exercises you can perform, as will one with a high number of

adjustment levels. Make sure that the bench is comfortable to lie on when you're lifting a heavy weight and that you can set it at a height that allows you to lie with your back and shoulders on the bench and both feet flat on the floor.

A bench-press bench with adjustable arms that hold the bar will be useful for doing heavy standing exercises such as squats and shoulder presses – unless you have a friend with you at all times – because they allow you to raise the bar safely.

Barbell

What it does

There are two main types of barbell: standard and Olympic. Standard ones use a spinlock system to secure the weight plates. Olympic bars use collars to secure the weight plates, have a two-inch diameter grip, which is broader than a standard bar, and come in either five, six or seven foot lengths. Full-length Olympic bars typically weigh 20kg, with shorter ones slightly less. Olympic bars can handle more weight and are sturdier than the standard option but are more expensive.

What to look for

The most important things to think about are the total weight of your plate set and the increments in which they ascend. If you want to do big compound lifts, such as squats, you will need a total weight that's at least equal to your bodyweight. But if you want to test yourself in the deadlift, that may need to rise to a set that's one and a half times your bodyweight.

Generally, the more precise you can be about the weight that you're lifting, the more chance you have of increasing

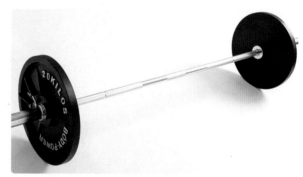

the amount you can lift. If you have a weight set that only goes up in 5kg increments you're going to struggle to get to the next level when

you want to increase your maximum lift because it's such a big jump. A set that includes 2.5kg and 1.25kg options will give you much more flexibility.

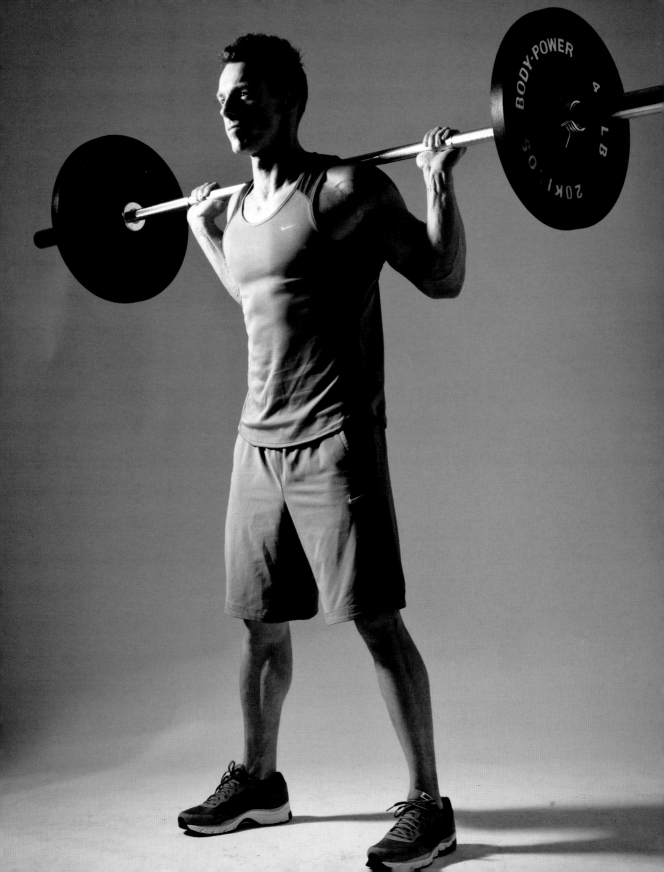

Barbell & bench I Exercises

01

Barbell curl

Target: biceps
Barbells allow you to up the load you lift for a biceps curl, shocking your muscles into new growth.

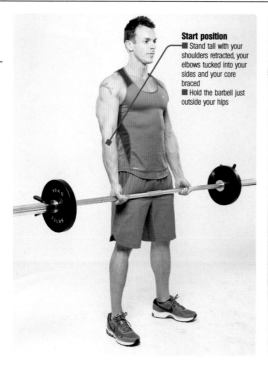

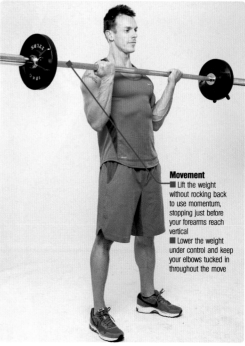

Start position
■ Stand tall with your shoulders retracted, your elbows tucked into your sides and your core braced
■ Hold the barbell just outside your hips

Movement
■ Lift the weight without rocking back to use momentum, stopping just before your forearms reach vertical
■ Lower the weight under control and keep your elbows tucked in throughout the move

02

Barbell rollout

Target: core
Engage your abs and your lower back to stabilise your core. The further you roll the bar, the harder the move becomes.

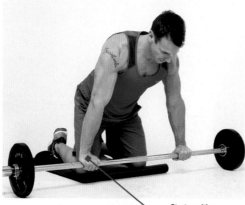

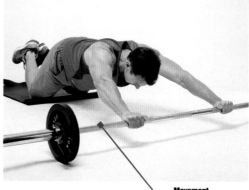

Start position
■ Start on your knees, holding the bar just wider than shoulder-width apart and directly beneath your shoulders

Movement
■ Keeping your back and arms straight and your core braced, roll the bar out in front of you
■ Stop before you feel you'll lose form and return the way you came

Fit Tip

Push yourself further

Once you get good at doing this move with barbell you can make it harder by doing the exercise with dumb-bells and alternately rowing them into your chest after rolling them out.

Exercises **|** Barbell & bench

Start position
■ Start with your core braced, your back straight and your shoulder blades retracted
■ Lean forward from the hips, rather than the waist, with your knees slightly bent
■ Grip the bar just wider than shoulder-width apart, letting the bar hang down around knee level

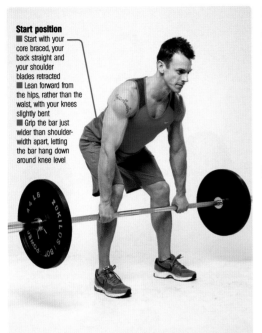

Movement
■ Pull the barbell up into your sternum, squeezing your shoulder blades together at the top of the move, then lower the bar slowly to the start

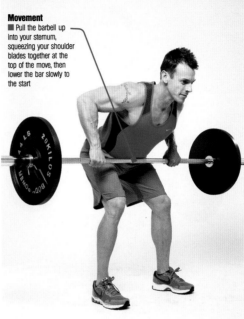

03

Bent-over row

Target: traps, lats, rhomboids
Use this big-muscle move to develop your back and give balance to the work you do on the bench press.

Start position
■ Start with your core braced, your back straight and your shoulder blades retracted
■ Lean forward from the hips, rather than the waist, and bend your knees slightly
■ Take an overhand grip just wider than shoulder width apart, letting the bar hang down around knee level

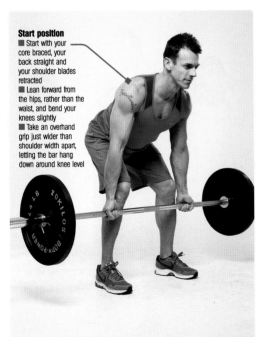

Movement
■ Pull the barbell up into your sternum, squeezing your shoulder blades together at the top of the move, then lower the bar slowly to the start

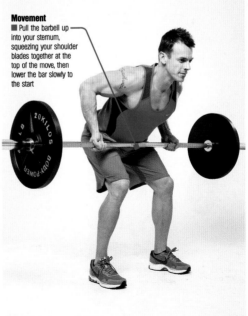

04

Reverse grip bent-over row

Target: traps, lats, rhomboids
Switch to a reverse grip to place more of an emphasis on your lats and lower traps.

Barbell & bench | Exercises

Shrug

Target: upper traps

Doing this move will increase your shoulder girdle stability, reducing your chances of injuring yourself during shoulder workouts.

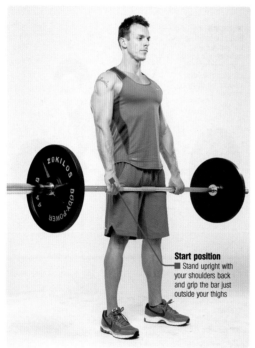

Start position
■ Stand upright with your shoulders back and grip the bar just outside your thighs

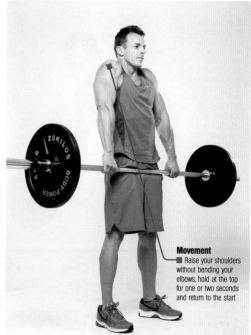

Movement
■ Raise your shoulders without bending your elbows, hold at the top for one or two seconds and return to the start

Upright row

Target: upper traps, shoulders

Hit both your traps and your shoulders with this simple move that develops vertical pulling strength. It's also a useful move to practice explosively before you move on to the more challenging hang clean.

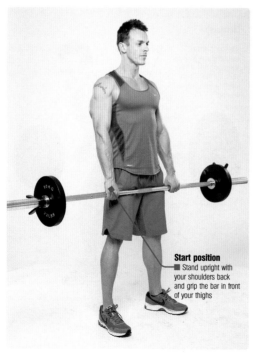

Start position
■ Stand upright with your shoulders back and grip the bar in front of your thighs

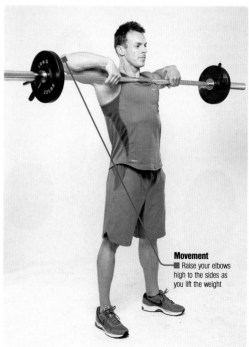

Movement
■ Raise your elbows high to the sides as you lift the weight

Exercises **| Barbell & bench**

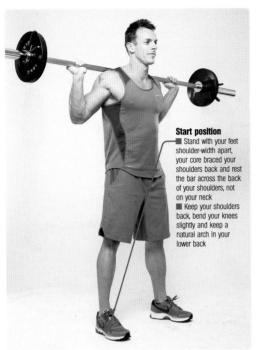

Start position
■ Stand with your feet shoulder-width apart, your core braced your shoulders back and rest the bar across the back of your shoulders, not on your neck
■ Keep your shoulders back, bend your knees slightly and keep a natural arch in your lower back

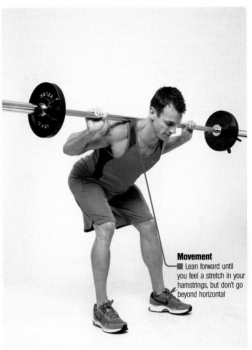

Movement
■ Lean forward until you feel a stretch in your hamstrings, but don't go beyond horizontal

07

Good morning

Target: lower back, hamstrings, glutes
This move will strengthen your middle back as well as your glutes and hamstrings but you'll need to maintain perfect form to avoid injury.

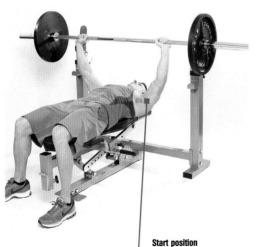

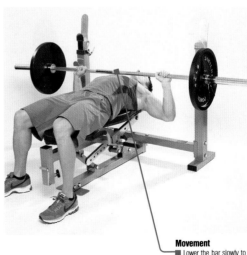

Start position
■ Rest your head and shoulders on the bench, brace your core, contract your shoulder blades and keep a natural arch in your spine
■ Bend your knees at 90˚ and keep your feet flat on the floor
■ Grip the bar with your hands just wider than shoulder-width apart, lift it from the rack and hold it directly above your chest

Movement
■ Lower the bar slowly to your chest and press back up powerfully
■ Press down with your feet to aid the movement but avoid arching your back during the pressing motion

08

Bench press

Target: chest
This classic test of strength will help you build a muscular chest.

Barbell & bench **I** Exercises

09

Incline bench press

Target: upper chest, front shoulder, triceps

Tilt the back support of the bench to hit your chest from a new angle and work your front shoulders and triceps.

Start position
■ Set the bench at 30-45°, brace your core and keep your feet flat on the floor
■ Grip the bar with hands slightly wider than shoulder-width apart
■ Remove the bar from the rack and hold the bar directly above your chest

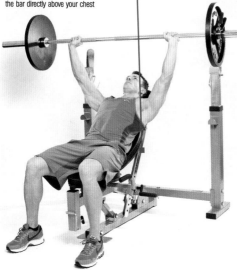

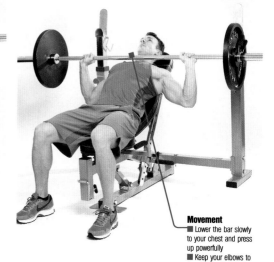

Movement
■ Lower the bar slowly to your chest and press up powerfully
■ Keep your elbows to the sides and don't arch your back

10

Decline bench press

Target: lower chest

Change the angle of the bench again to make sure you give your chest a balanced workout.

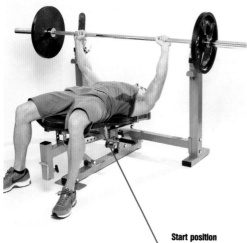

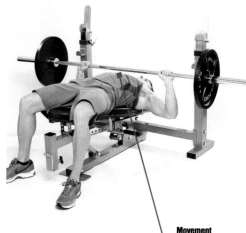

Start position
■ Set the bench at a decline
■ Grip the bar slightly wider than shoulder width apart, lift it from the rack and hold it directly above your chest

Movement
■ Lower the bar slowly to your chest and press back up powerfully
■ Keep your elbows to the sides and don't arch your back

Exercises | Barbell & bench

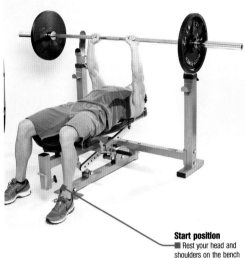

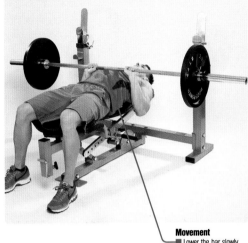

11

Close grip bench press

Target: triceps, chest
By bringing your hands closer together on the bench press, you transfer the emphasis of the exercise to your triceps.

Start position
■ Rest your head and shoulders on the bench and plant your feet flat on the floor
■ Brace your core and avoid arching your back
■ Keep your hands close together on the bar and squeeze your shoulder blades together

Movement
■ Lower the bar slowly towards your sternum, keeping your elbows tucked in, then press back up powerfully

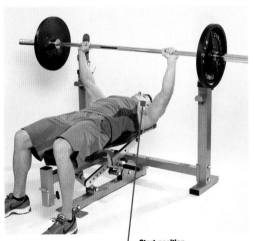

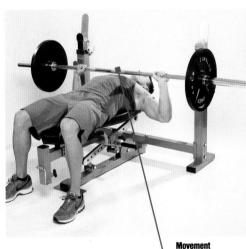

12

Ballistic bench press

Target: chest
Push the bar up explosively as if you were going to throw it to activate your fast-twitch muscle fibres. Just remember to hang on to the bar.

Start position
■ Rest your head and shoulders on the bench, brace your core, contract your shoulder blades and keep a natural arch in your spine
■ Bend your knees at 90° and keep your feet flat on the floor
■ Grip the bar with your hands just wider than shoulder-width apart, lift it from the rack and hold it directly above your chest

Movement
■ Lower the bar slowly to your chest and press back up as quickly as you can while maintaining control
■ Press down with your feet to aid the movement but avoid arching your back during the pressing motion

Barbell & bench I Exercises

13

Squat

Target: quads, glutes, hamstrings
This must-do lower-body move will flood your body with muscle growth hormones and improve your body's ability to stabilise itself.

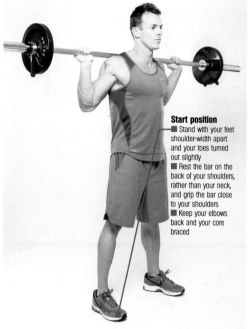

Start position
- Stand with your feet shoulder-width apart and your toes turned out slightly
- Rest the bar on the back of your shoulders, rather than your neck, and grip the bar close to your shoulders
- Keep your elbows back and your core braced

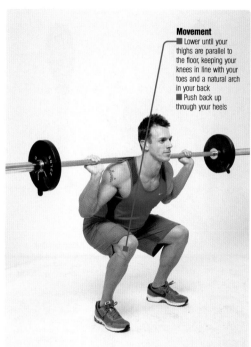

Movement
- Lower until your thighs are parallel to the floor, keeping your knees in line with your toes and a natural arch in your back
- Push back up through your heels

14

Jump squat

Target: quads, glutes, hamstrings
Add a jump to your squat to add a plyometric element to your workout.

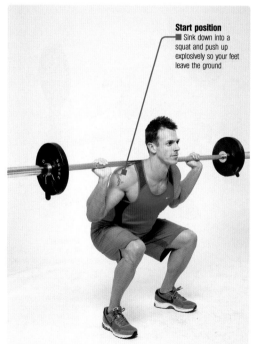

Start position
- Sink down into a squat and push up explosively so your feet leave the ground

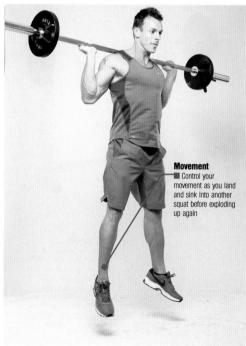

Movement
- Control your movement as you land and sink into another squat before exploding up again

Exercises | Barbell & bench

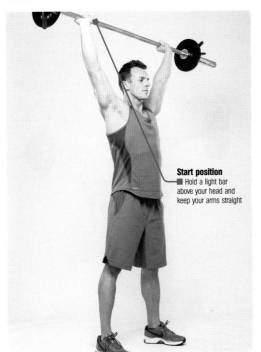

Start position
■ Hold a light bar above your head and keep your arms straight

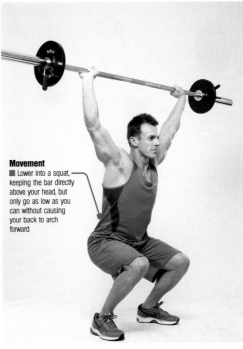

Movement
■ Lower into a squat, keeping the bar directly above your head, but only go as low as you can without causing your back to arch forward

15

Overhead squat

Target: quads, glutes, hamstrings
Performing the move with the weight above your head tests your posture because poor shoulder mobility will force the weight forward as you squat down.

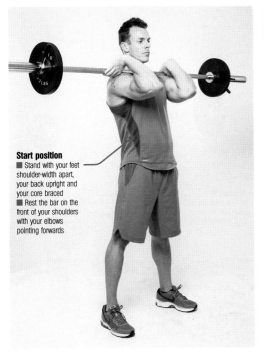

Start position
■ Stand with your feet shoulder-width apart, your back upright and your core braced
■ Rest the bar on the front of your shoulders with your elbows pointing forwards

Movement
■ Lower until your thighs are parallel to the floor, keeping your knees in line with your toes and your elbows as high as you can
■ Push back up powerfully through your heels

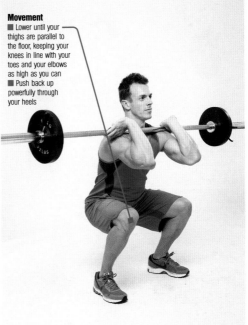

16

Front squat

Target: quads
Placing the bar on the front of your shoulders forces your back to be more upright and shifts the emphasis onto your quads and away from your lower back.

Barbell & bench **|** Exercises

17

Lunge

Target: glutes, hamstrings, quads

Boost your power and coordination with this classic functional lower-body move.

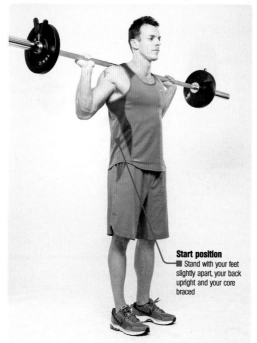

Start position
■ Stand with your feet slightly apart, your back upright and your core braced

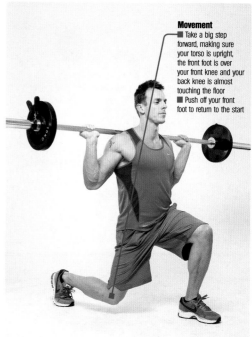

Movement
■ Take a big step forward, making sure your torso is upright, the front foot is over your front knee and your back knee is almost touching the floor
■ Push off your front foot to return to the start

18

Split squat

Target: quads, glutes, hamstrings

This move is like a lunge but you start with one foot forward, which is less of a coordination test but allows you to lift heavier weights than a standard lunge.

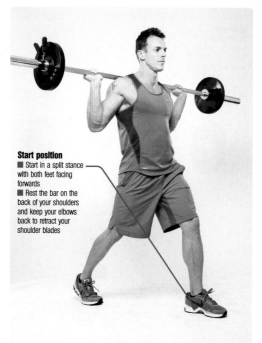

Start position
■ Start in a split stance with both feet facing forwards
■ Rest the bar on the back of your shoulders and keep your elbows back to retract your shoulder blades

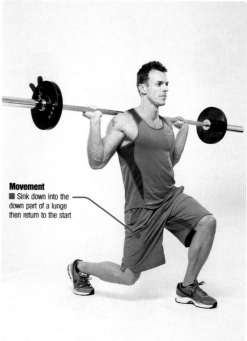

Movement
■ Sink down into the down part of a lunge then return to the start

Exercises | Barbell & bench

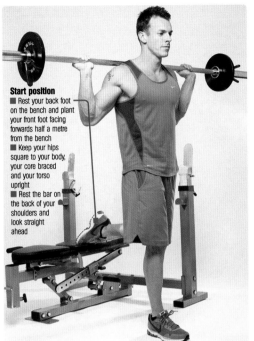

Start position
- Rest your back foot on the bench and plant your front foot facing forwards half a metre from the bench
- Keep your hips square to your body, your core braced and your torso upright
- Rest the bar on the back of your shoulders and look straight ahead

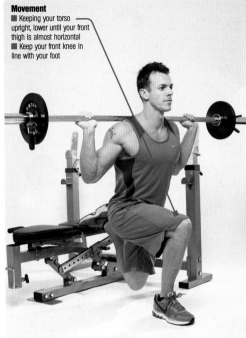

Movement
- Keeping your torso upright, lower until your front thigh is almost horizontal
- Keep your front knee in line with your foot

19

Bulgarian split squat

Target: quads, glutes
Placing your back foot on the bench concentrates all the effort onto the front foot, giving you a unilateral workout and balanced muscle gain.

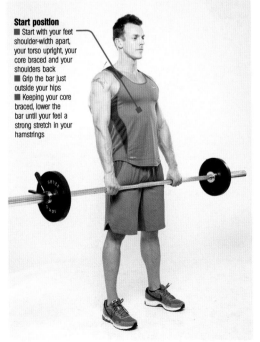

Start position
- Start with your feet shoulder-width apart, your torso upright, your core braced and your shoulders back
- Grip the bar just outside your hips
- Keeping your core braced, lower the bar until your feel a strong stretch in your hamstrings

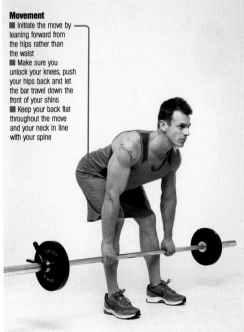

Movement
- Initiate the move by leaning forward from the hips rather than the waist
- Make sure you unlock your knees, push your hips back and let the bar travel down the front of your shins
- Keep your back flat throughout the move and your neck in line with your spine

20

Romanian deadlift

Target: hamstrings
Use this move to make sure you get balanced muscle growth if your workouts include quad-dominant squats. It's also great for teaching your back, hips and legs to work together.

Barbell & bench I Exercises

21

Stiff-legged Romanian deadlift

Target: hamstrings

Keeping your legs straight increases the challenge to your hamstrings but can put stress on your lower back so start light and use perfect form.

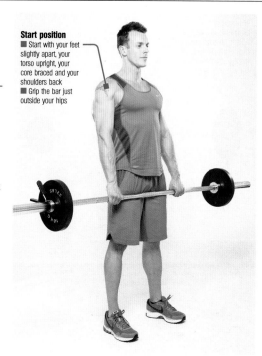

Start position
■ Start with your feet slightly apart, your torso upright, your core braced and your shoulders back
■ Grip the bar just outside your hips

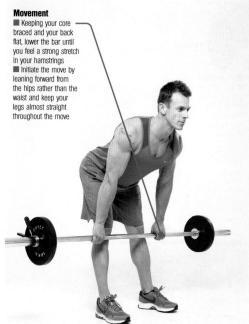

Movement
■ Keeping your core braced and your back flat, lower the bar until you feel a strong stretch in your hamstrings
■ Initiate the move by leaning forward from the hips rather than the waist and keep your legs almost straight throughout the move

22

Shoulder press

Target: deltoids

This must-do move will add strength and size to your shoulders.

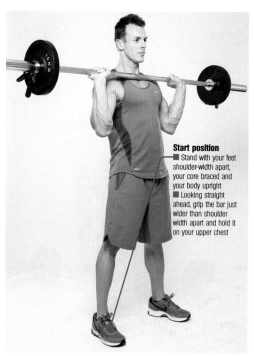

Start position
■ Stand with your feet shoulder-width apart, your core braced and your body upright
■ Looking straight ahead, grip the bar just wider than shoulder width apart and hold it on your upper chest

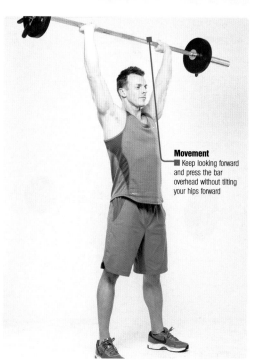

Movement
■ Keep looking forward and press the bar overhead without tilting your hips forward

Exercises ▮ Barbell & bench

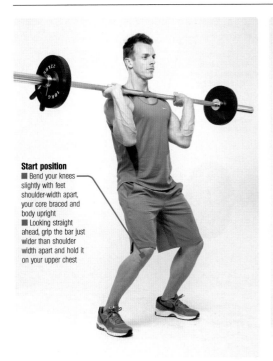

Start position
■ Bend your knees slightly with feet shoulder-width apart, your core braced and body upright
■ Looking straight ahead, grip the bar just wider than shoulder width apart and hold it on your upper chest

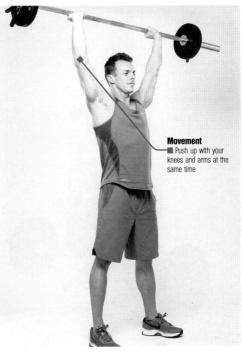

Movement
■ Push up with your knees and arms at the same time

23

Push press

Target: deltoids
Use your legs to initiate the move, which will allow you to press more weight and will improve your dynamic pushing power.

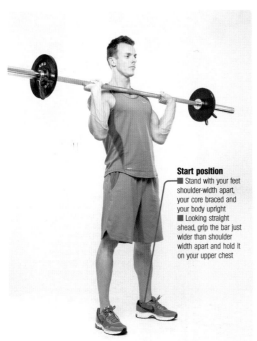

Start position
■ Stand with your feet shoulder-width apart, your core braced and your body upright
■ Looking straight ahead, grip the bar just wider than shoulder width apart and hold it on your upper chest

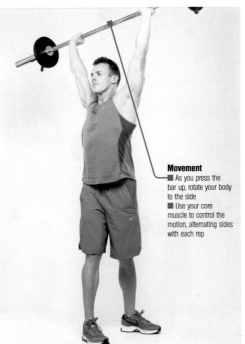

Movement
■ As you press the bar up, rotate your body to the side
■ Use your core muscle to control the motion, alternating sides with each rep

24

Shoulder press with rotation

Target: deltoids, core
Work your shoulders and core simultaneously by calling on your midsection to control the rotation.

Barbell & bench I Exercises

Deadlift

Target:
quads, glutes, hamstrings, back, core

This is one of the most effective muscle-building moves you can do.

Start position
■ Start with your feet shoulder-width apart and hold the bar close to your shins with an overhand or alternate grip just outside your knees
■ Look forward, brace your core and position your shoulders over the bar, keeping your back flat and your shoulders retracted

Movement
■ Start the lift by pushing with your glutes and pushing down through your heels
■ Keeping your shoulders back, the bar should rise up your shins
■ As the bar passes your knees, push your hips forward

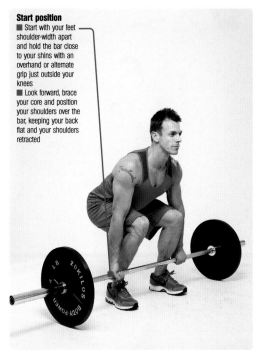

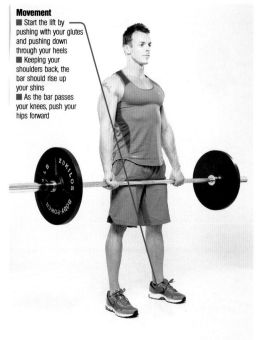

Clean & jerk

Target:
whole body

This Olympic lift hits virtually every muscle in your body, for an explosive, challenging workout.

Start position
■ Start in a deadlift position

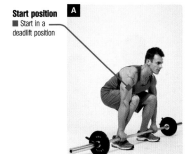

A

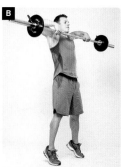

B

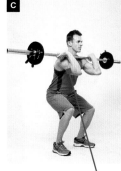

C

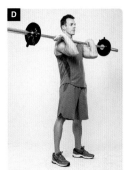

D

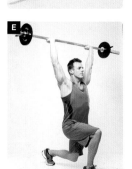

E

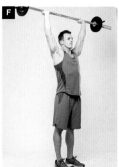

F

Movement
■ Pull the bar explosively to your chest, keeping your elbows high and rising up onto your toes to gain power
■ Bend your knees to duck under the bar at its highest point, flipping the bar onto your fingers and catching it on top of your chest
■ Stand up straight to steady yourself then drop into a lunge, simultaneously pressing the bar overhead
■ Stand up straight to complete the move

Exercises | Barbell & bench

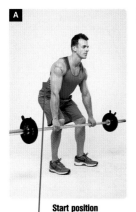

A

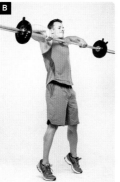

B

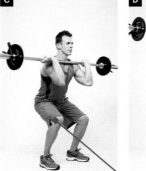

C

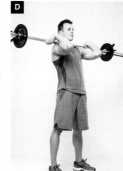

D

27

Hang clean

**Target:
hamstrings,
glutes, calves,
back, shoulders**
This dynamic
whole-body move
will develop power
and trains your
body to generate
force efficiently.

Start position
■ Start with your feet
shoulder-width apart, your
core braced and your back
straight
■ Grip the bar just
outside your knees and
lean forward slightly from
the hips

Movement
■ Bend your knees to
initiate the move and pull
the bar up powerfully to your
chest, keeping your elbows
high and rising up onto your
toes to gain power
■ Bend your knees to duck
under the bar at its highest
point, flipping the bar onto
your fingers and catching it
on top of your chest
■ Stand up straight
and reset the bar before
repeating

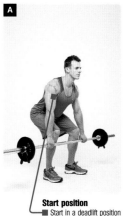

A

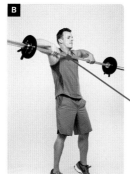

B

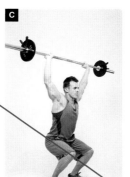

C

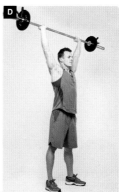

D

28

Snatch

**Target: whole
body**
The other Olympic
lift develops total-
body strength and
power production.
It requires high
levels of technique
and concentration
so pay attention to
your form.

Start position
■ Start in a deadlift position

Movement
■ Pull the bar explosively
to your chest, keeping
your elbows high and
rising up onto your toes to
gain power
■ Duck beneath the bar to
catch it with straight arms,
keeping your back in its
natural arch
■ Stand up straight before
resetting the bar and
repeating the move

Fit Tip

Stand tall

Before doing any big lift, imagine
reaching towards the ceiling with
the top of your head to correct your
posture and lift your shoulders.

Barbell & bench I **Exercises**

29

Romanian deadlift to row

Target: glutes, hamstring, back
Work the big muscles at the back of your body with this classic combination exercise.

A

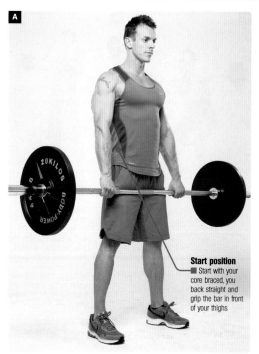

Start position
- Start with your core braced, you back straight and grip the bar in front of your thighs

B

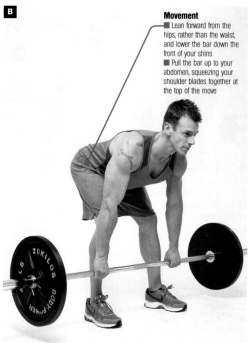

Movement
- Lean forward from the hips, rather than the waist, and lower the bar down the front of your shins
- Pull the bar up to your abdomen, squeezing your shoulder blades together at the top of the move

C

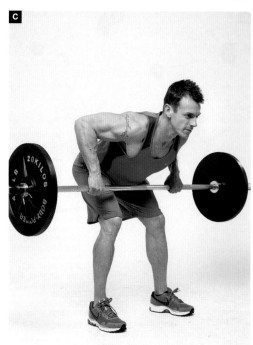

Full-body workout

Full-body workouts allow you to work a large number of muscle fibres in one session. They should involve multi-joint moves that hit several muscle groups at once and flood the body with growth hormones. They're also a good option if you're new to training because they get your muscles used to weight training without putting them under too much stress.

The downside of a full-body workout is that it's hard to fully exhaust your muscle fibres when using this method, so you may want to also do some more muscle-specific sessions (which are explained in this section).

Designing your workout

The most important thing in a full-body routine is balance. You need an equal number of pushing and pulling movements and you should spend roughly the same amount of time on your upper and lower body. Using compound exercises (multi-joint moves that work several muscle groups at once) will give you the best training effect.

Leave abs exercises to the end of your workout because you don't want to exhaust your core muscles before they're called upon to stabilise your spine in more demanding moves such as the squat or the pull-up.

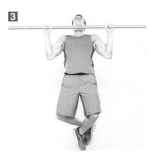
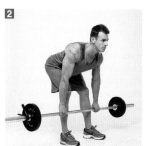
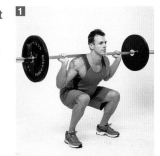
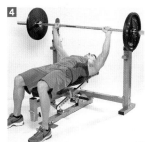
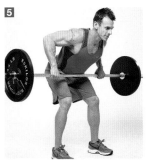
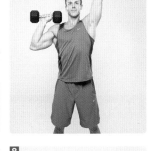
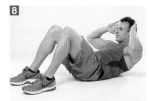
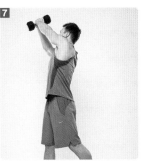

Full-body sample workout

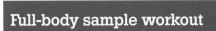

1 Barbell squat | **Sets:** 3 **Reps:** 10-12 **Page:** 142

2 Romanian deadlift | **Sets:** 3 **Reps:** 10-12 **Page:** 145

3 Pull-up | **Sets:** 3 **Reps:** to failure **Page:** 107

4 Bench press | **Sets:** 3 **Reps:** 10-12 **Page:** 139

5 Bent-over row | **Sets:** 3 **Reps:** 10-12 **Page:** 137

6 Alternating dumb-bell shoulder press
Sets: 3 **Reps:** 10-12 **Page:** 75

7 Woodchop | **Sets:** 2 **Reps:** 10 each side **Page:** 82

8 Crunch | **Sets:** 3 **Reps:** 15 **Page:** 27

Barbell & bench I **Workouts**

Body focus workout

While full-body workouts let you work a big range of muscle fibres, the advantage of body focus workouts is that you can completely fatigue the target muscles. You can then let them recover for a week while you train different body parts. It's a good way of being specific about how you put on muscle but the downside is that doing lots of single-joint exercises won't produce as big a growth hormone release as doing big compound moves. You also need to be prepared to exercise frequently to work every major muscle group once a week.

Designing your workout
The structure of your session is particularly important if you're doing a body focus routine because you want to train the target muscle hard but without overtraining or risking injury.

Start by doing light exercises that will warm up your joint before moving on to do the bigger muscle-building moves. You must then make sure you have fully fatigued the muscle by doing a single-joint move. Vary the exercises and angles you use to work your target body part so that you get good balanced muscle growth.

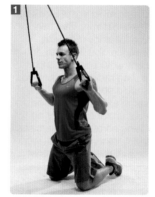

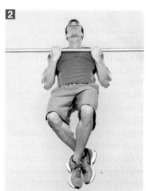

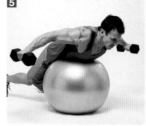

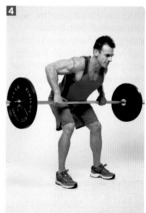

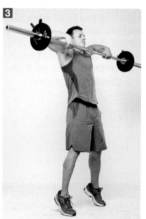

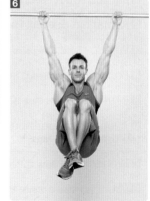

Body focus sample workout:
upper back and lats

1 Lat pull down I **Sets: 2 Reps: 10 Page: 120**

2 Chin-up I **Sets: 2 Reps: to failure Page: 106**

3 Hang clean I **Sets: 2 Reps:10 Page: 149**

4 Barbell bent-over row I **Sets: 2 Reps: 10 Page: 137**

5 Gym ball dumb-bell reverse flye I **Sets: 2 Reps: 10 Page: 63**

6 Hanging knee raise I **Sets: 2 Reps: 10 Page: 108**

Workouts I Barbell & bench

Core stability workout

Good core stability is absolutely essential if you want to lift heavy weights, be better at sport and stay injury free. Your core muscles are the ones around your midriff, including your abdominals and lower back, and their function is to provide a link between your upper and lower body. They're particularly important during whole-body moves, which need a strong core to transfer power between the upper and lower halves of your body. They're also called upon to stabilise your spine during dynamic and sporty movements.

A weak core will inhibit your ability to lift heavy weights in whole-body moves because you won't be able to transfer force from your lower to upper body. You may also get lower back or postural problems.

Developing your workout
To get a strong and stable midsection you need to attack your core from different angles and target the muscles at the sides and back of your midriff. Using a range of items of kit will help you achieve that because they challenge your muscle in different ways.

Start with moves that place most weight on your core, such as compound lifts, and end with bodyweight exercises that won't risk injuring your tired muscles. Because this workout focuses on stability, complete a relatively high number of reps per set.

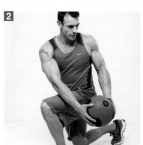

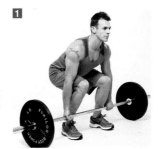

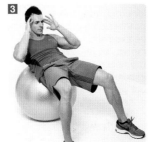

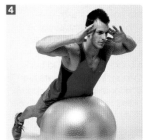

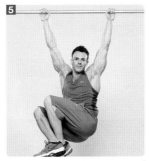

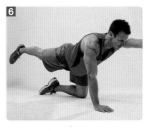

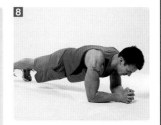

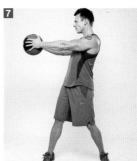

Core stability sample workout

1 Deadlift I **Sets: 3 Reps: 10-12 Page: 148**

2 Medicine ball lunge chop I **Sets: 2 Reps: 15 Page: 111**

3 Gym ball crunch I **Sets: 2 Reps: 15 Page: 57**

4 Gym ball back extension **Sets: 2 Reps: 15 Page: 62**

5 Twisting knee raise I **Sets: 2 Reps: 12 each side Page: 110**

6 Two-point box I **Sets: 2 Reps: 15 each side Page: 33**

7 Tornado chop I **Sets: 2 Reps: 15 each side Page: 116**

8 Plank I **Sets: 1 Time: hold as long as possible Page: 29**

Barbell & bench I Workouts

Circuit training workout

Circuit workouts can be very tiring because you don't rest between exercises. For that reason, people often choose to use comparatively light weights such as dumb-bells or medicine balls. That doesn't, however, mean you can't use a barbell – it just means that you shouldn't use a weight that will cause you to fatigue too early.

Approach your circuit in the same way you would when using other bits of kit. Perform the exercises back to back to keep your effort level high and force your heart to pump blood to different parts of your body for both a cardiovascular and a muscle-building benefit.

Designing your workout
For circuits to be effective, you need to move from one exercise to the next as swiftly as possible. Using a barbell for every exercise will help you do this.

Pick a group of exercises that target as many different muscle groups as possible and alternate between upper and lower body moves to make your heart work harder without experiencing excessive muscle fatigue. Include a good mix of pushing, pulling, lunging, bending and rotational moves, to give your workout balance. You should also try to complete the reps quickly but without compromising good form.

Once you have completed the circuit, rest for three minutes, then do it all again. The fitter you become the more circuits you'll be able to complete.

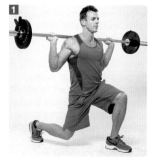

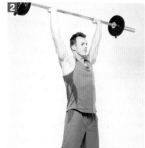

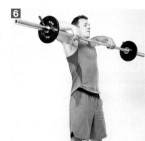

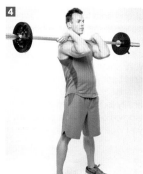

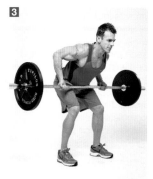

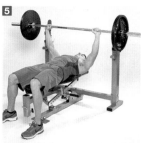

Circuit training sample workout

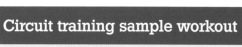

1 Lunge I **Sets: 1 Reps: 10 each side Page: 144**

2 Shoulder press I **Sets: 1 Reps: 10 Page: 146**

3 Reverse-grip bent-over row I **Sets: 1 Reps: 10 Page: 137**

4 Front squat I **Sets: 1 Reps: 10 Page: 143**

5 Bench press I **Sets: 1 Reps: 10 Page: 139**

6 Hang clean I **Sets: 1 Reps: 6 Page: 149**

7 Barbell rollout I **Sets: 1 Reps: 10 Page: 136**

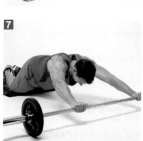

Explosive power workout

Explosive power workouts, also known as plyometric workouts, give you more than one typeof benefit. They help build muscle but also develop your power and coordination. During a plyometric move, you activate the muscle eccentrically as it's stretched out and pre-loaded, then you explode into the lift to contract the muscle concentrically, which shortens it.

This dynamic movement targets your fast-twitch muscle fibres, exhausting them quicker then a conventional workout but without having to add extra weight. The intensity will also push up your heart rate, burning extra calories and releasing muscle-building hormones into your body.

This method of workout are popular with sportsmen because they develop fast, movements and improve skills such as jump distance..

Designing your workout

The intensity and force generated during explosive power workouts means that they carry a slightly higher injury risk. For that reason, you should perform fewer repetitions of each plyometric exercise than you would for a standard workout. For the plyometric moves, use a weight that's 30-40 per cent of your ten-rep maximum for that exercise.

For each target body part, start by doing an activation move to warm-up and stabilise your muscles. Then do the plyometric exercise before performing a single-joint move to exhaust the muscles.

The emphasis of these sessions is on speed and power, rather than developing endurance, rest for at least one minute between plyometric sets and at least two minutes between plyometric exercises.

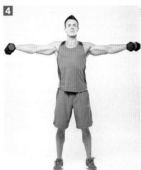
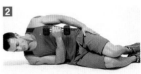
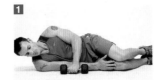
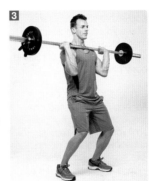
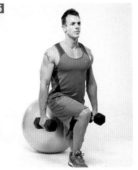
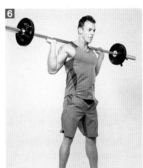
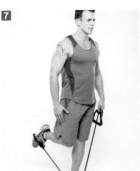

Plyometric sample workout:
shoulders and legs

1 External dumb-bell rotation I **Sets: 3 Reps: 10 Page: 80**

2 Internal dumb-bell rotation I **Sets: 3 Reps: 10 Page: 80**

3 Push press I **Sets: 3 Reps: 8 Page: 147**

4 Lateral raise I **Sets: 2 Reps: 10 each side Page: 77**

5 Split dumb-bell Romanian deadlift
Sets: 2 Reps: 10 each side Page: 71

6 Jump squat I **Sets: 3 Reps: 6 Page: 142**

7 Resistance band leg curl I **Sets: 2
Reps: 10 each side Page: 122**

Barbell & bench I Workouts

Superset workout

A superset workout will let you work a huge number of muscles in relatively short period of time because you do two exercises back to back before resting.

Any two exercises can be paired together to form a superset but the most popular option, and the one we've selected for the workout opposite, is to create 'antagonistic supersets', where the two moves work opposing body parts. An example would be to perform an incline bench press (which works your upper chest), then go straight into a bent-over row (which works your back). The advantage of antagonistic supersets is that they give one body part a chance to rest while the opposing muscle group is

working to ensure balanced muscle development.

Other common forms include non-competing supersets, which target unrelated muscle groups, such as pairing a lower-body move with an upper-body one, and post-exhaustion supersets, where you do a multi-joint move followed by a single-joint move targeting the same body part.

Designing your workout

For each exercise, find one that works its polar opposite, so if you do one exercise that targets your quads do another that targets your hamstrings. Biceps exercises should be paired with triceps moves, and so on. After each superset, rest for two minutes and repeat.

1 Superset A

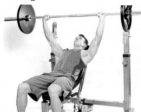
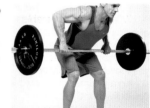

2 Superset B

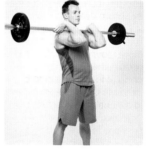
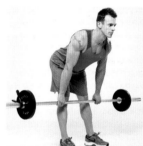

3 Superset C

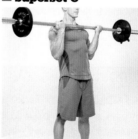
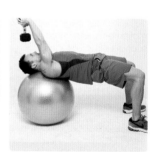

4 Superset D

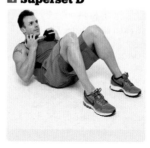
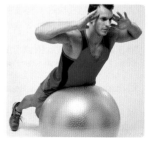

Superset sample workout

1 Superset A

Incline bench press I Bent-over row
Sets: 3 **Reps:** 10-12 **Page:** 140, 137

2 Superset B

Front squat I Stiff-legged deadlift
Sets: 3 **Reps:** 10-12 **Page:** 143, 146

3 Superset C

Barbell curl I Lying triceps extension
Sets: 3 **Reps:** 10-12 **Page:** 136, 55

4 Superset D

Dumb-bell crunch I Gym ball back extension
Sets: 3 **Reps:** 10-12 **Page:** 57, 62

Body part split workout

As you become more advanced, you may find that you're unable to sufficiently fatigue your muscles in a full-body routine. If that's the case, you should consider doing a split routine where you do a different thing in each session of the week. The most popular form of split routine is a body part split where you train two body parts in a single session. An example of this would be to train your legs and back in your first workout of the week, your chest and triceps in the second, your shoulders and biceps in the third and you abs and core in the fourth. This system lets you hit every body part hard once a week

without having to go to the gym every day.

Designing your workout
Once you have decided on which two body parts you're going to work, do a move that works one of these body parts then alternate between the two body parts. So, for example, if you're going to work your legs and back you could start with a Romanian deadlift, which works your hamstrings, then do a good morning, which targets your back. To fully develop the body part, make sure you include a range of exercises that hit the target muscle groups from a variety of angles.

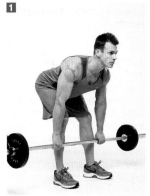

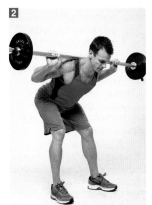

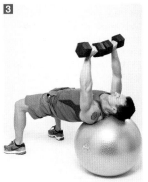

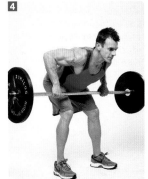

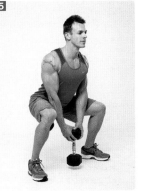

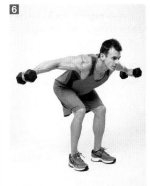

Body part split sample workout: legs and back

1 Romanian deadlift I **Sets:** 3 **Reps:** 10-12 **Page:** 145

2 Good morning I **Sets:** 3 **Reps:** 10-12 **Page:** 139

3 Gym ball dumb-bell chest press
Sets: 3 **Reps:** 10-12 **Page:** 64

4 Bent-over row I **Sets:** 3 **Reps:** 10 **Page:** 137

5 Sumo squat I **Sets:** 3 **Reps:** 10 **Page:** 68

6 Dumb-bell bent over flye I **Sets:** 2 **Reps:** 10 **Page:** 62

Barbell & bench I Workouts

Upper/lower body split workout

Splitting your routines into either upper or lower body sessions is an easy way to arrange your workouts. It may be tempting to do more upper-body sessions but try to keep the split even, otherwise you'll end up with a muscular torso and scrawny legs.

This type of workout is attractive because it's simple to create so you don't have to spend lots of time planning your sessions. They also suit people who can't fit in many sessions per week because you only have to do two sessions a week to make sure you've worked every major muscle group. You will, however, need to do more than two sessions a week if you want to see the best benefits.

Designing your workout
If you're doing a lower-body day, all of your exercises should target your lower body. To make sure your routine is balanced, you should include moves that work your glutes, quads, hamstrings and calves. You should also try to hit them from different angles. Start with the biggest muscles such as your quads and hamstrings then do calves moves.

If you're doing an upper-body workout, the same principles apply so you'd work your chest, back and shoulders before targeting the smaller muscles of your biceps, triceps and forearms.

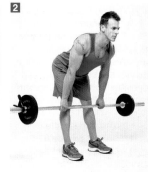

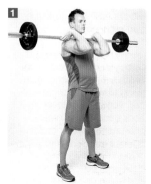

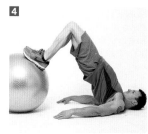

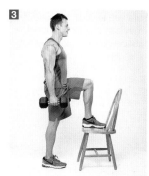

Upper/lower body split sample workout: lower body

1 Front squat I **Sets:** 3 **Reps:** 10-12 **Page:** 143

2 Stiff-legged Romanian deadlift
Sets: 3 **Reps:** 10-12 **Page:** 146

3 Dumb-bell step-up I **Sets:** 2 **Reps:** 10 each side **Page:** 70

4 Gym ball leg curl I **Sets:** 3 **Reps:** 10 **Page:** 72

5 Supine gym ball calf raise I **Sets:** 3 **Reps:** 10-12 **Page:** 74

6 Wall squat I **Sets:** 1 **Time:** hold as long as possible **Page:** 39

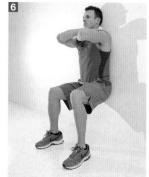

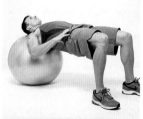

Workouts | Barbell & bench

Push/pull split workout

A push/pull split routine is similar to an upper lower/body one in that you do two types of workout. In this case, you alternate between workouts involving pushing moves and workouts involving pulling moves. This way of splitting workouts can be attractive for people who do sports that involve a lot of pushing movements, such as rugby, because it focuses your sessions around those kinds of movements. You still, however, need to do an equal amount of pulling moves to make sure you get balanced muscle development.

Designing your workout

If you're doing a pull day, all the moves in your workout should be pulling moves. Pulling moves are ones that work your back, hamstrings, biceps and abs. Aim to make your workout balanced, so include moves that work all of those body parts and use different exercises and angles in different push sessions. Do moves that target big muscles such as your back and hamstrings, then go on to the smaller muscles of your biceps and abs. If you're doing a pushing workout, the same rules apply.

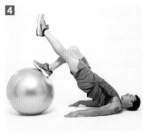
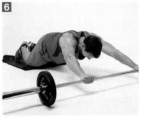
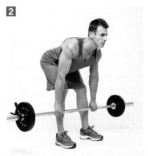
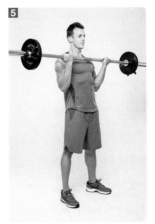
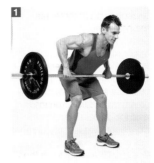
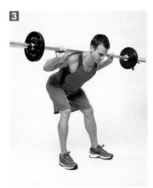

Push/pull split sample workout: pull session

1 Bent-over row | **Sets:** 3 **Reps:** 10-12 **Page:** 137

2 Romanian deadlift | **Sets:** 3 **Reps:** 10-12 **Page:** 145

3 Good morning | **Sets:** 3 **Reps:** 10-12 **Page:** 139

4 One-leg gym ball hamstring curl
Sets: 2 **Reps:** 10 each side page **Page:** 73

5 Barbell curl | **Sets:** 3 **Reps:** 10-12 **Page:** 136

6 Barbell rollout | **Sets:** 3 **Reps:** 10-12 **Page:** 136

Barbell & bench I **Workouts**

Post-exhaustion workout

A s we saw in the dumb-bell and gym ball section, weight training exercises can be divided into two main categories – compound moves and isolation moves. Compound exercises use several muscle groups at once while isolation exercises target one muscle group on its own. Post-exhaustion training involves pairing a compound move with an isolation one.

Designing your workout

In post-exhaustion workouts, the compound move always comes first. The theory is that you do a big muscle move to get yourself pumped by moving heavy weights. then you move on to the lighter weight isolation move to completely fatigue the target muscle.

If you're training your back, you could do a bent-over row, for example, which recruits your lats, traps and rhomboids. You could then do a bent-over reverse dumb-bell flye, which works your upper back.

You must avoid doing the isolation move first because this may fatigue your target muscle. When you come to lift the heavy weight of a compound move your smaller stabilising muscles will be under increased strain, which can increase your chances of injury.

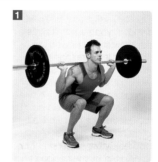

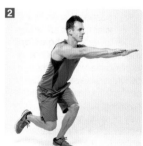

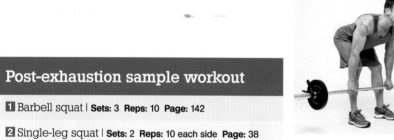

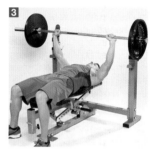

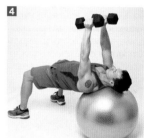

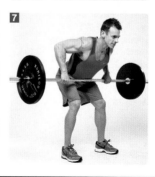

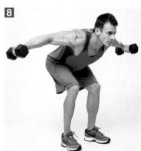

Post-exhaustion sample workout

1 Barbell squat I **Sets:** 3 **Reps:** 10 **Page:** 142

2 Single-leg squat I **Sets:** 2 **Reps:** 10 each side **Page:** 38

3 Bench press I **Sets:** 3 **Reps:** 10 **Page:** 139

4 Gym ball dumb-bell flye I **Sets:** 3 **Reps:** 12 **Page:** 66

5 Romanian deadlift I **Sets:** 3 **Reps:** 10 **Page:** 145

6 Gym ball hamstring curl I **Sets:** 3 **Reps:** 12 **Page:** 72

7 Bent-over row I **Sets:** 3 **Reps:** 10 **Page:** 137

8 Bent-over dumb-bell flye I **Sets:** 3 **Reps:** 12 **Page:** 62

Pyramid workout

Essentially, pyramid workouts involve increasing the weight that you lift with each set of an exercise while reducing the number of reps you perform. This is good because there's no such thing as a slightly activated muscle fibre – they are either engaged completely or not at all. By taking a muscle through an increasing range of weight while reducing the reps, you target each category of fibres in turn, completely exhausting the whole muscle.

Designing your workout

Doing a whole workout of pyramid exercises would take a long time and could be counter-productive, overtraining the muscle and sending the body into a destructive metabolism. Instead, strategically inserting pyramid sets into a workout will give you all the benefits of this method.

There is more than one way of performing a pyramid workout. One way, which is outlined below, is to start with a conventional muscle growth rep count, such as ten, and reduce the number of reps you do by two each set until you get to four reps. You can also include a reverse pyramid by starting with low reps and ending with a high rep count.

You can adjust your rep counts depending on what you want to achieve. If your focus is on strength, start with fewer reps and go down to as little as one rep for a set. You can also gradually reduce your reps before gradually increasing them so you finish with the same number of reps you completed for your first set.

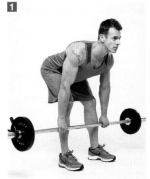

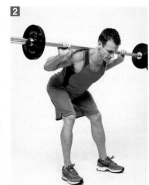

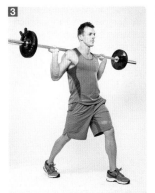

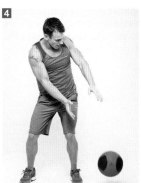

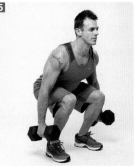

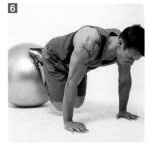

Pyramid sample workout:
legs and core

1 Romanian deadlift
Sets: 4 Reps: Pyramid 10/8/6/4 **Page: 145**

2 Good morning | **Sets: 3 Reps: 10 Page: 139**

3 Split squat | **Sets: 2 Reps:** 10 each side **Page: 144**

4 Medicine ball throw downs
Sets: 2 Reps: 10 each side **Page: 114**

5 Dumb-bell squat | **Sets: 3 Reps: 10 Page: 67**

6 Gym ball jackknife
Sets: 4 Reverse pyramid 4/6/8/10 Page: 59

Barbell & bench **I** Workouts

Drop set workout

D
rop sets are a way of increasing the number of reps you perform of an exercise. Once you reach failure on your final set of an exercise, immediately reduce the weight and do as many reps as you can with that weight. Once you reach failure again, drop the weight once more and continue that process.

The intense nature of this system ramps up the muscle-building effect so use them to iron out weak muscle links. To do them effectively and to minimise the time between reaching failure and starting the new weight, you may want to use a training partner to help you adjust the weights.

Designing your workout
Drop sets are a demanding technique so use them

sparingly. Make sure that you only do them on the final set of the final exercise of a body part because they completely exhaust the muscle involved. If you tried to do more exercises for that body part you would struggle to use perfect form.

For the same reason, you should only perform one or two drop sets per workout. Do more and you risk overtraining. You can use as many drops as you like, provided you maintain strict form. Make sure you drop the weight at increments that have a positive but not too dramatic an effect on how many reps you can perform. Dropping the weight by 20 per cent is a good place to start. If you halve the weight you won't take full advantage of the technique's muscle-building potential.

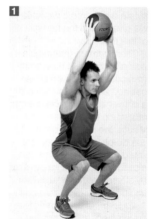
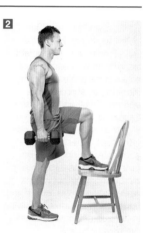
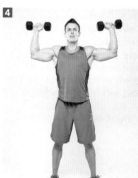
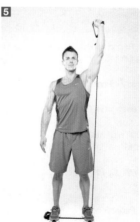
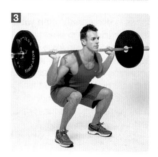
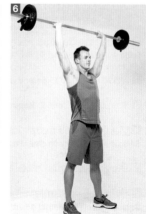

Drop set sample workout:
legs and shoulders

1 Med ball overhead squat **I Sets: 3 Reps: 10 Page:** 117

2 Dumb-bell step-up **I Sets: 2 Reps: 10 each side Page:** 70

3 Squat **I Sets: 3 (last set drop set) Reps:** 10-12 **Page:** 142

4 Cuban press **I Sets: 3 Reps:** 10-12 **Page:** 78

5 One-arm resistance band shoulder press
Sets: 3 Reps: 10 Page: 120

6 Barbell shoulder press
Sets: 3 (last set drop set) Reps: 10-12 **Page:** 146

Workouts **| Barbell & bench**

Back-off set workout

Back-off sets involve doing between 2-4 sets of low reps with a heavy weight of an exercise before dropping the weight significantly for a final set where you do as many reps as possible.

The reason this is effective is because the nerves that stimulate your muscles are primed for action by the heavy sets, allowing you to perform better in the final set than you would had you attempted that set before the heavy sets. This increased capacity sparks new muscle growth.

Designing your workouts

For a back-off set to work, it has to be a move that you can do using heavy weights and one that you can control how much weight you're lifting. That's why big compound moves such as a bench press, rather than stability or

bodyweight exercises work best for back-off sets.

You'll get best results by activating the target muscle group before working it again in a back-off exercise. When you come to do your back off exercise, choose a weight that you could lift six times. When you do the back-off set, drop the weight by 40 per cent and do as many reps as you can while maintaining perfect form. If, for example, you ordinarily lift 50kg on the bench press, reduce this to 30kg for the back-off set.

Aim to perform the reps of a back-off set faster than you would during a regular set to simultaneously develop your explosive power and your strength. This way of working out can be very draining so only use it sparingly to challenge your muscles. Do it for one week as part of a six-to-eight-week programme.

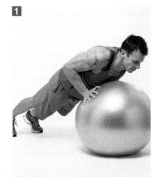

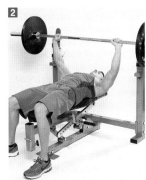

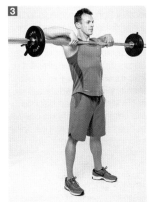

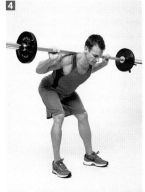

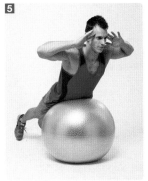

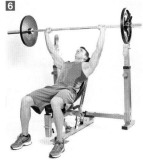

Back-off set sample workout:
chest and back

1 Gym ball press-up **| Sets:** 3 **Reps:** 10 **Page:** 65

2 Bench press **| Sets:** 3 (+1 back off set)
Reps: 6 (+ as many as you can in back off set) **Page:** 139

3 Upright row **| Sets:** 3 **Reps:** 10 **Page:** 138

4 Good morning **| Sets:** 3 (+1 back off set)
Reps: 6 (+ as many as you can in back off set) **Page:** 139

5 Gym ball back extension **| Sets:** 3 **Reps:** 10 **Page:** 62

6 Incline bench press **| Sets:** 3 (+1 back off set)
Reps: 6 (+ as many as you can in back off set) **Page:** 140

Barbell & bench **I Workouts**

Wave-loading workout

There are a number of ways that you can do a wave-loading session but, essentially, they all involve lifting a weight for a set then cutting the reps but upping the weight for the next set. From here you can either go back to the original weight and perform as many reps as you can or reduce the reps and up the weight for another set before repeating that sequence of three sets.

Whatever way you decide to arrange your wave-loading workout, the method teaches your muscles to lift more weight in a single rep so it"s a good tool to use if you're struggling to increase your maximum lift for an exercise.

Designing your workout
Wave-loading workouts work well in split routines because you can activate the body part with a stability move before wave loading for the strength move and fully exhausting the target muscle in an isolation move.

One option for wave-loading moves is to find your five-rep maximum for an exercise, then do four reps. Rest for three minutes, increase the weight by five per cent then do three reps. Rest for three minutes, increase the weight by five per cent and do two reps. Rest for three minutes and repeat the process.

An alternative, and the one outlined in the sample workout on this page, is to do a normal set of eight reps then rest for two minutes before loading extra weight onto your dumb-bells for a shorter set of four reps. Another rest of two minutes is followed by a final set in which you go back to the original weight and crank out as many reps as possible, taking you past eight reps.

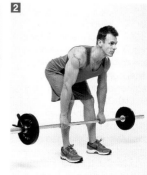
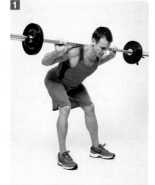
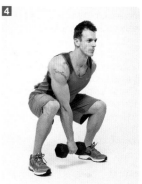
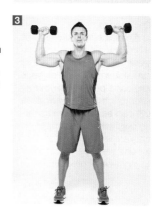
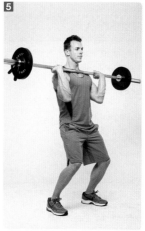
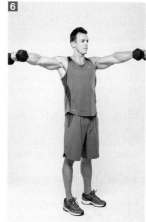

Wave-loading sample workout

1 Good morning | **Sets:** 3 **Reps:** 10-12 **Page:** 139

2 Romanian deadlift | **Sets:** 3
Reps: (wave loader) 8, 4, 8+ **Page:** 145

3 Cuban press | **Sets:** 3 **Reps:** 10-12 **Page:** 78

4 Single-arm dumb-bell snatch | **Sets:** 2
Reps: 10 each side **Page:** 81

5 Barbell push press | **Sets:** 3
Reps: (wave loader) 8, 4, 8+ **Page:** 147

6 Front/lateral raise | **Sets:** 3 **Reps:** 10-12 **Page:** 78

Cluster workout

Cluster workouts are a good way of injecting new stimulus into your workouts. There are a number of ways of doing cluster workouts but essentially they all involve reducing the load so you can cut your rest times. The result is that you lift a greater volume of weight in a session, which has a positive effect on muscle growth and calorie burn.

Designing your workout

One of the simplest ways to do a cluster workout is to do a normal workout until you get to the final two exercises. If you have done ten reps for each move, stick with a weight that you'd use to do ten reps for the final two moves if you were continuing your standard workout but only do five reps of the penultimate exercise.

Without resting, move on to the final exercise and do five reps. Go straight back to the penultimate exercise and alternate between the final two moves for five minutes, doing five reps of each without resting. Make sure you chose opposing or non-competing muscle groups such as legs and back, otherwise you'll fatigue early.

Other ways of doing cluster workouts include doing single reps with your three rep maximum with minimal rest between reps (ten seconds, say) or clusters of low rep sets of one exercise with your ten rep maximum using minimal rest between groups of reps. However you choose to arrange your workouts, this is an intense method so use it when you feel your progress has stalled.

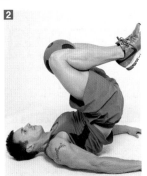

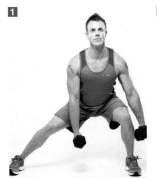

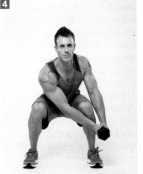

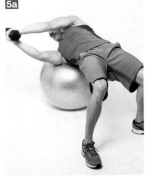

Cluster sample workout

1 Side lunge | **Sets:** 2 **Reps:** 10 each side **Page:** 69

2 Medicine ball reverse crunch
Sets: 3 **Reps:** 10 **Page:** 112

3 Deadlift | **Sets:** 3 **Reps:** 10 **Page:** 148

4 Dumb-bell woodchop
Sets: 2 **Reps:** 10 each side **Page:** 82

5a Gym ball Russian twist | **Clusters** 1 **Reps:** 5 **Page:** 61

5b Good morning | **Clusters** 1 **Reps:** 5 **Page:** 139

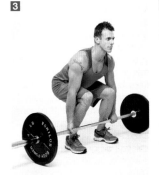

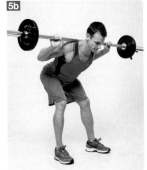

Home gym I Machines

Home gym machines guide

If you have the space and funds, home gym machines can help to improve your fitness

Cardio machines

Doing cardio workouts will improve an important aspect of your fitness. It is possible to get a cardio effect from weight training, as we've seen in the sample circuit workouts in each kit chapter. But if you really want to improve your cardio ability, and enter races, you could benefit from buying a cardio machine.

The main types of cardio machine are treadmills, stationary bikes and rowing machines. You can of course run and cycle outside, and both of those activities are fantastic at improving your cardio fitness, but a machine is a convenient weather-immune option. And unless you live near a lake and have access to boats, an indoor rower is also probably going to be more convenient.

If you decide to buy a piece of cardio equipment you'll be confronted by a bewildering array of options, ranging from bargain products to ones that cost the same as a small car. What you go for depends on your budget and your exercise goals but, whatever your funds and aspirations, this section will give you the knowledge needed to make the right choice. We've also given you three different types of cardio session to try for each type of kit.

If you do get a cardio machine, avoid doing the same session over and over again. You'll soon get bored and stop improving. In the same way that you need to keep challenging your muscles if you want to get bigger and stronger, you need to make sure you vary your

cardio training if you want to become aerobically fitter.

Multigyms

The quality of home multigyms has improved enormously in recent years. The best ones now mimic the movements you make when using freeweights, which allows you to push yourself without getting trapped under a heavy barbell. They're also increasingly space efficient.

The cheaper options will lock you into fixed planes of motion, so it's the machine, rather than your muscles, that controls a large part of the movement. More sophisticated (and, therefore, expensive) machines may either have cables, where movement patterns aren't fixed, or the option to switch between fixed path and freeweights.

What is cardio?

Cardio fitness essentially refers to your body's ability to generate energy through the circulation of blood and oxygen. You can improve your cardio fitness by doing aerobic exercise, which is any activity that you can sustain for more than a few minutes that requires your heart and lungs to work harder in order to meet your body's demand for oxygen. Running, cycling and rowing will all increase your cardio fitness, helping you to exercise for longer and burn more calories, as well as improving your heart and lung function.

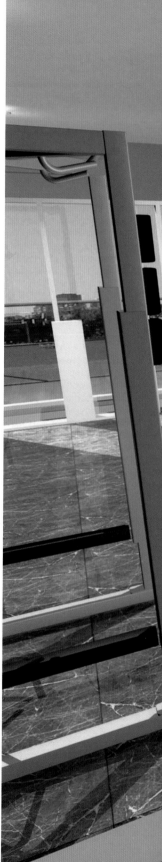

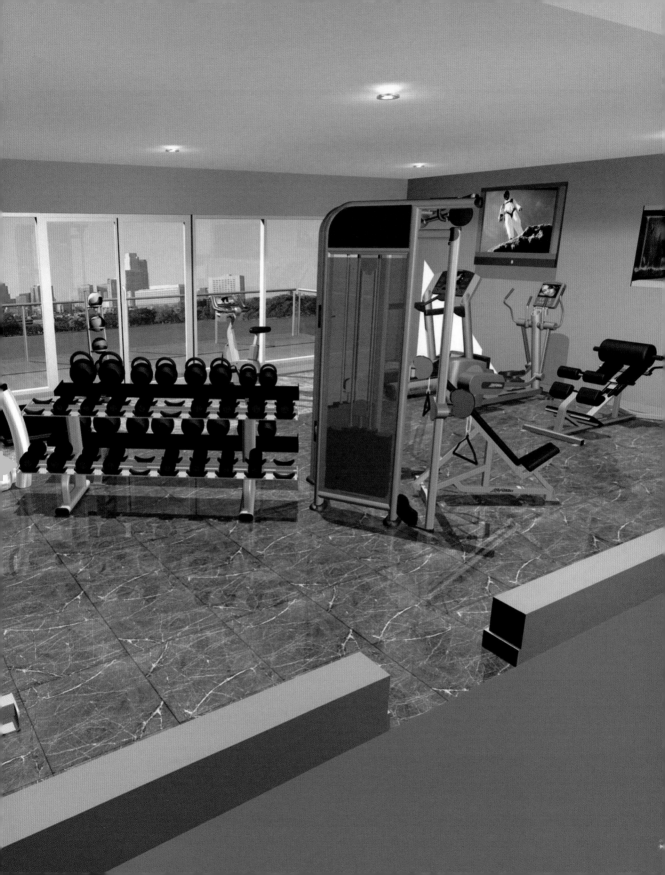

Home gym I Machines

How to buy... a rowing machine

WHY GET ONE?

Rowing with proper form will work all your major muscle groups as well as being excellent low-impact cardiovascular exercise (compared to running on a pavement, which is high impact because it hammers your joints). Top-quality rowers are generally cheaper than other bits of cardio kit too, so you can get a serious workout without having to spend excessive sums of money.

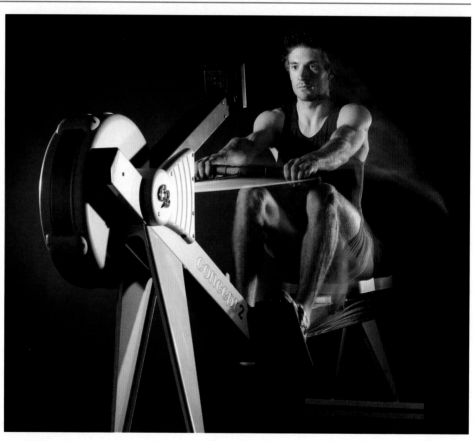

Rowing workouts

Do these sessions to get fit and stay motivated

Stroke intervals

Row at an easy pace for a few minutes to warm up, reset the counter then find a stroke rate that puts you at a slightly harder pace for five minutes. Then explode into action, increasing your stroke rate by five to ten strokes per minute and hold this rate for 60 seconds. Drop back down to the previous stroke rate for five minutes and increase it by five to ten again for another 60 seconds. Repeat once more to complete your workout.

500s

Do 500m to warm up, then reset the counter. Accelerate into the next 500m and note the time that you achieve. Then recover for 500m. Accelerate for another 500m and try to beat your previous time. Continue this pattern for 20 minutes, trying to make each interval faster than the last.

Rowing pyramids

Warm up for five minutes then row for two minutes at a pace of 26 strokes per minute. Increase the stroke rate every two minutes until you get to 32 strokes per minute before working back down to 26 per minute. Then do five hard rows followed by five easy rows. Repeat but increase the rows by five each time until you get to 25 before working back down to five. Warm down by rowing at an easy pace for five minutes.

Machines I Home gym

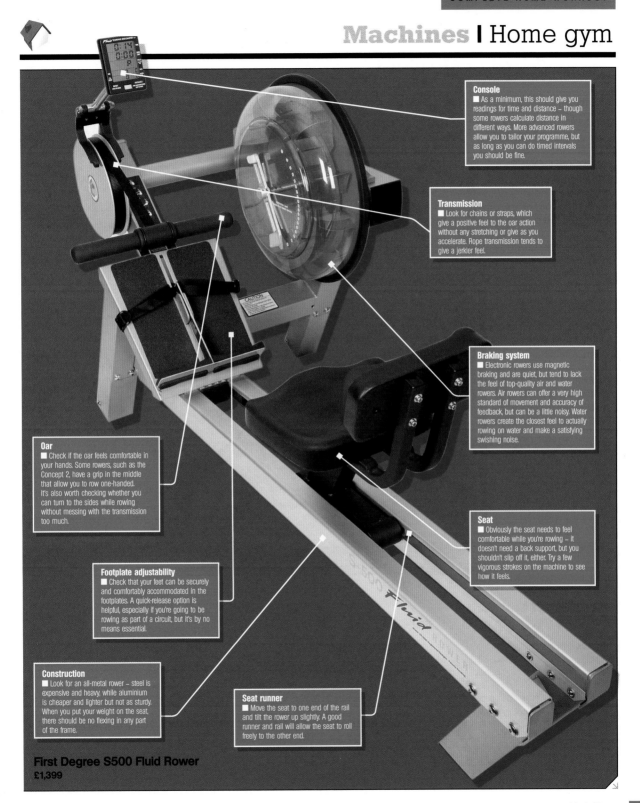

Console
■ As a minimum, this should give you readings for time and distance – though some rowers calculate distance in different ways. More advanced rowers allow you to tailor your programme, but as long as you can do timed intervals you should be fine.

Transmission
■ Look for chains or straps, which give a positive feel to the oar action without any stretching or give as you accelerate. Rope transmission tends to give a jerkier feel.

Braking system
■ Electronic rowers use magnetic braking and are quiet, but tend to lack the feel of top-quality air and water rowers. Air rowers can offer a very high standard of movement and accuracy of feedback, but can be a little noisy. Water rowers create the closest feel to actually rowing on water and make a satisfying swishing noise.

Oar
■ Check if the oar feels comfortable in your hands. Some rowers, such as the Concept 2, have a grip in the middle that allow you to row one-handed. It's also worth checking whether you can turn to the sides while rowing without messing with the transmission too much.

Seat
■ Obviously the seat needs to feel comfortable while you're rowing – it doesn't need a back support, but you shouldn't slip off it, either. Try a few vigorous strokes on the machine to see how it feels.

Footplate adjustability
■ Check that your feet can be securely and comfortably accommodated in the footplates. A quick-release option is helpful, especially if you're going to be rowing as part of a circuit, but it's by no means essential.

Construction
■ Look for an all-metal rower – steel is expensive and heavy, while aluminium is cheaper and lighter but not as sturdy. When you put your weight on the seat, there should be no flexing in any part of the frame.

Seat runner
■ Move the seat to one end of the rail and tilt the rower up slightly. A good runner and rail will allow the seat to roll freely to the other end.

First Degree S500 Fluid Rower
£1,399

Home gym | Machines

How to buy... a treadmill

WHY GET ONE?

A treadmill has traditionally been one of the pricier bits of home gym kit, but recently the quality models have dropped in price enough to become an attractive option. They're an excellent form of cardio, and make running a more pleasant option in rainy weather. And they'll give your knees a bit of a break from pounding the pavements.

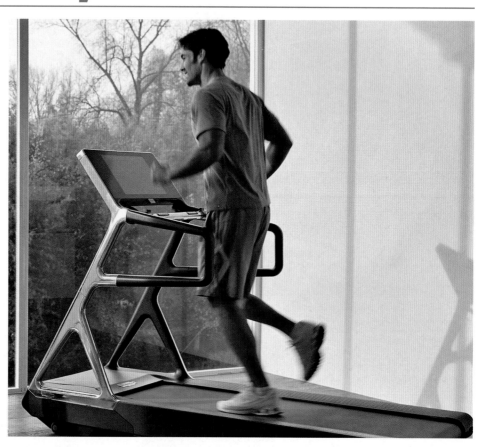

Treadmill training

Plodding is boring so try these challenging 20-minute workouts

Pack of cards

Take a pack of cards with you to the treadmill. Jog and then do a progressive, five-minute warm-up. Stop and turn over a card, then run for one minute at the effort level of the card – one is walking pace and nine is the top speed you can sustain for 60 seconds.

If you get a ten or a picture card, sprint for as long as possible up to 30 seconds. Do this for 20 minutes.

Negative split

Do a five-minute progressive warm-up. Then reset the timer and do seven minutes at level 6-7 (using the 'Pack of cards' effort scale). After seven minutes raise the speed so that you're running at level 7-8. Try to hold that pace for another eight minutes. Running faster in the second half of a race is a tactic known as a negative split, and this session will maximise the training effect and teach you good race strategy.

Hill running

Jog for five minutes, then run up a 'hill' at level 6-7 (again, using the 'Pack of cards' effort scale) for one minute by setting the treadmill incline to eight per cent, then reset the incline and jog for a minute. Go back to an eight per cent incline and sprint at level 8-9, so you cover the same distance in 30-40 seconds before removing the incline. Keep alternating this pattern for a total of 12 hill reps. Jog for a couple of minutes to warm down.

Machines | Home gym

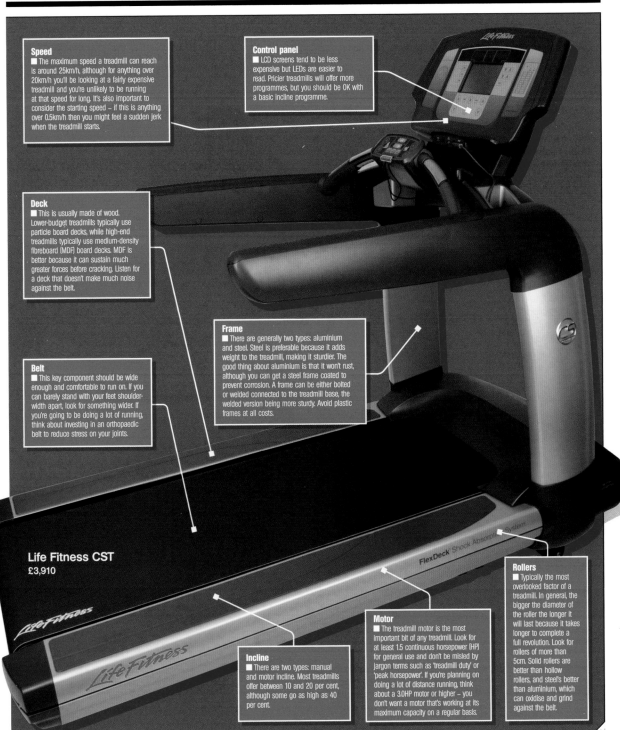

Speed
■ The maximum speed a treadmill can reach is around 25km/h, although for anything over 20km/h you'll be looking at a fairly expensive treadmill and you're unlikely to be running at that speed for long. It's also important to consider the starting speed – if this is anything over 0.5km/h then you might feel a sudden jerk when the treadmill starts.

Control panel
■ LCD screens tend to be less expensive but LEDs are easier to read. Pricier treadmills will offer more programmes, but you should be OK with a basic incline programme.

Deck
■ This is usually made of wood. Lower-budget treadmills typically use particle board decks, while high-end treadmills typically use medium-density fibreboard (MDF) board decks. MDF is better because it can sustain much greater forces before cracking. Listen for a deck that doesn't make much noise against the belt.

Frame
■ There are generally two types: aluminium and steel. Steel is preferable because it adds weight to the treadmill, making it sturdier. The good thing about aluminium is that it won't rust, although you can get a steel frame coated to prevent corrosion. A frame can be either bolted or welded connected to the treadmill base, the welded version being more sturdy. Avoid plastic frames at all costs.

Belt
■ This key component should be wide enough and comfortable to run on. If you can barely stand with your feet shoulder-width apart, look for something wider. If you're going to be doing a lot of running, think about investing in an orthopaedic belt to reduce stress on your joints.

Life Fitness CST
£3,910

FlexDeck Shock Absorption System

Rollers
■ Typically the most overlooked factor of a treadmill. In general, the bigger the diameter of the roller the longer it will last because it takes longer to complete a full revolution. Look for rollers of more than 5cm. Solid rollers are better than hollow rollers, and steel's better than aluminium, which can oxidise and grind against the belt.

Motor
■ The treadmill motor is the most important bit of any treadmill. Look for at least 1.5 continuous horsepower (HP) for general use and don't be misled by jargon terms such as 'treadmill duty' or 'peak horsepower'. If you're planning on doing a lot of distance running, think about a 3.0HP motor or higher – you don't want a motor that's working at its maximum capacity on a regular basis.

Incline
■ There are two types: manual and motor incline. Most treadmills offer between 10 and 20 per cent, although some go as high as 40 per cent.

Home gym I Machines

How to buy... an exercise bike

WHY GET ONE?

The engineering required to build a quality exercise bike is less expensive than the equivalent in a decent treadmill, so you can get a good cardio workout for relatively little cash. Working out on a bike is easier on the knees than running – and if you've got any history of lower-back problems, a recumbent will be much better for you than a rowing machine.

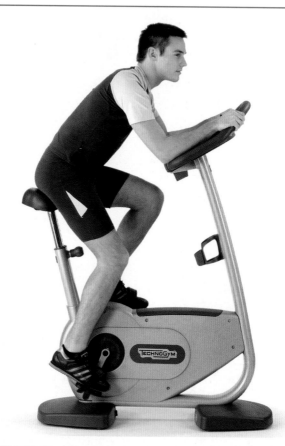

Bike workouts

Try these stationary bike sessions to inject life into your riding

Speedy spinning

Do a five-minute warm-up. Cycle at level 6-7 (where 1 is walking pace and 9 in the top speed you could sustain for one minute) for two minutes and then explode into motion, pedalling as fast as you possibly can. Lean forward on the handlebars and let your legs fly for 20-30 seconds. Make a note of the top RPM that you reach. Rest for 30 seconds and then go back to pedalling at level 6-7 for one minute before repeating the effort. Do this ten times in total.

Test lactic acid resistance

Warm up for five minutes at level 4-5 (using the 'Speedy spinning' effort scale). Now accelerate until you're working at level 8 so that you can feel your legs start to burn with lactic acid but you're not forced to slow down. Hold this pace for five minutes and then drop back to level 4-5 for two minutes. Accelerate back up to level 8 for five minutes, then select a low resistance and spin your pedals for three minutes to flush the lactic acid out of your muscles.

More resistance, same cadence

Cycle at an easy pace for five minutes, then increase the resistance of your pedals without reducing your cadence. Continue cycling with that level of resistance before going back to the easier resistance level for two minutes. Repeat that four times and warm down with five minutes easy cycling.

Machines I Home gym

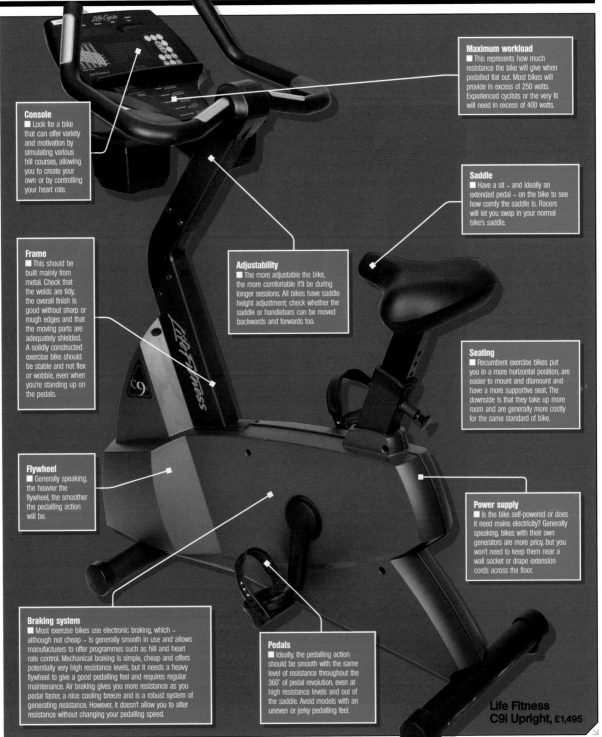

Maximum workload
■ This represents how much resistance the bike will give when pedalled flat out. Most bikes will provide in excess of 250 watts. Experienced cyclists or the very fit will need in excess of 400 watts.

Console
■ Look for a bike that can offer variety and motivation by simulating various hill courses, allowing you to create your own or by controlling your heart rate.

Saddle
■ Have a sit – and ideally an extended pedal – on the bike to see how comfy the saddle is. Racers will let you swap in your normal bike's saddle.

Frame
■ This should be built mainly from metal. Check that the welds are tidy, the overall finish is good without sharp or rough edges and that the moving parts are adequately shielded. A solidly constructed exercise bike should be stable and not flex or wobble, even when you're standing up on the pedals.

Adjustability
■ The more adjustable the bike, the more comfortable it'll be during longer sessions. All bikes have saddle height adjustment; check whether the saddle or handlebars can be moved backwards and forwards too.

Seating
■ Recumbent exercise bikes put you in a more horizontal position, are easier to mount and dismount and have a more supportive seat. The downside is that they take up more room and are generally more costly for the same standard of bike.

Flywheel
■ Generally speaking, the heavier the flywheel, the smoother the pedalling action will be.

Power supply
■ Is the bike self-powered or does it need mains electricity? Generally speaking, bikes with their own generators are more pricy, but you won't need to keep them near a wall socket or drape extension cords across the floor.

Braking system
■ Most exercise bikes use electronic braking, which – although not cheap – is generally smooth in use and allows manufacturers to offer programmes such as hill and heart rate control. Mechanical braking is simple, cheap and offers potentially very high resistance levels, but it needs a heavy flywheel to give a good pedalling feel and requires regular maintenance. Air braking gives you more resistance as you pedal faster, a nice cooling breeze and is a robust system of generating resistance. However, it doesn't allow you to alter resistance without changing your pedalling speed.

Pedals
■ Ideally, the pedalling action should be smooth with the same level of resistance throughout the 360˚ of pedal revolution, even at high resistance levels and out of the saddle. Avoid models with an uneven or jerky pedalling feel.

**Life Fitness
C9i Upright, £1,495**

Home gym I Machines

How to buy... a multigym

WHY GET ONE?

Multigym production has come on in leaps and bounds over the last few years, with options on the market that mimic the benefits of free weights (such as instability) while letting you lift heavy without a spotter standing by. They're also more space-efficient these days, making it more plausible to keep one in the house without annoying other residents such as wives.

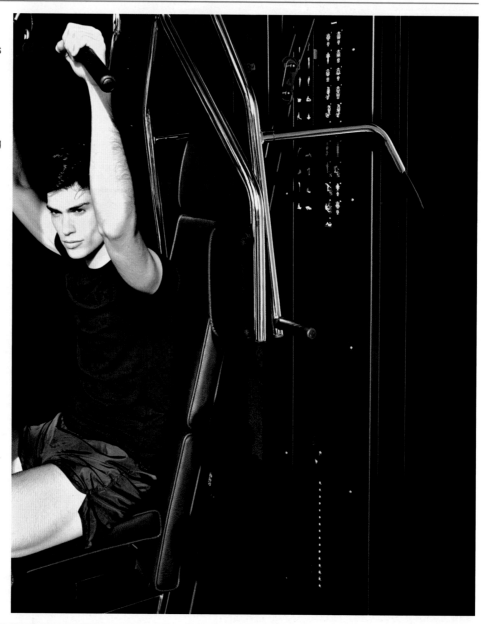

Machines | Home gym

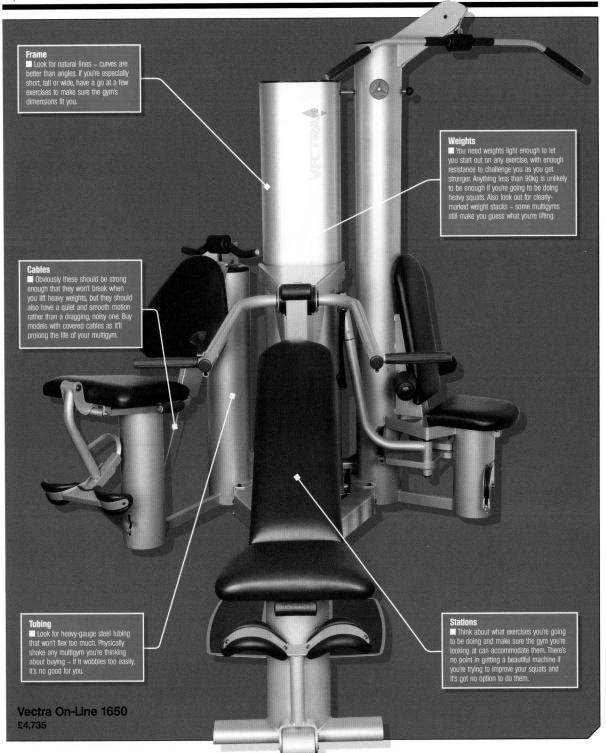

Frame
■ Look for natural lines – curves are better than angles. If you're especially short, tall or wide, have a go at a few exercises to make sure the gym's dimensions fit you.

Weights
■ You need weights light enough to let you start out on any exercise, with enough resistance to challenge you as you get stronger. Anything less than 90kg is unlikely to be enough if you're going to be doing heavy squats. Also look out for clearly-marked weight stacks – some multigyms still make you guess what you're lifting.

Cables
■ Obviously these should be strong enough that they won't break when you lift heavy weights, but they should also have a quiet and smooth motion rather than a dragging, noisy one. Buy models with covered cables as it'll prolong the life of your multigym.

Tubing
■ Look for heavy-gauge steel tubing that won't flex too much. Physically shake any multigym you're thinking about buying – if it wobbles too easily, it's no good for you.

Stations
■ Think about what exercises you're going to be doing and make sure the gym you're looking at can accommodate them. There's no point in getting a beautiful machine if you're trying to improve your squats and it's got no option to do them.

Vectra On-Line 1650
£4,735

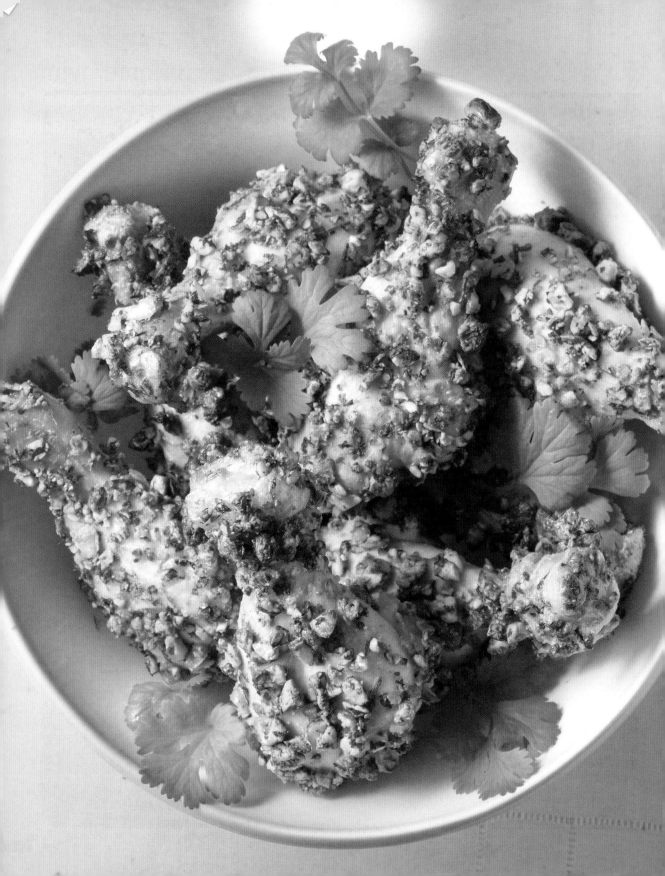

Introduction | Nutrition

Fuel your training

Make the most of your workouts by fuelling them with the right foods

The food you eat has a huge impact on the results you see from your workouts. Your body needs fuel for you to exercise effectively and the nutritional materials to repair your muscles so they get bigger. That's why your workouts will be wasted unless they're backed up by proper nutrition.

This section will explain the fundamentals of eating for more muscle. It also contains a sample meal plan that you can use to make sure you're taking on board the right kind of foods. We've also included a comprehensive guide to sports supplements, giving you the knowledge you need to decide whether or not you want to use them to complement your training.

The good news is that eating well doesn't involve going on fad diets or cutting out large food groups. In fact, you'll need to consume plenty of calories to power your workouts and build new muscle.

Wherever possible, you should eat fresh, unprocessed food. One simple rule to follow is that if people weren't eating it 1,000 years ago, then don't eat it now. Processed foods tend to be high in calories and low in nutritional value, so avoid them where you can. You should also eat a wide variety of foods to make sure you get enough vitamins and minerals.

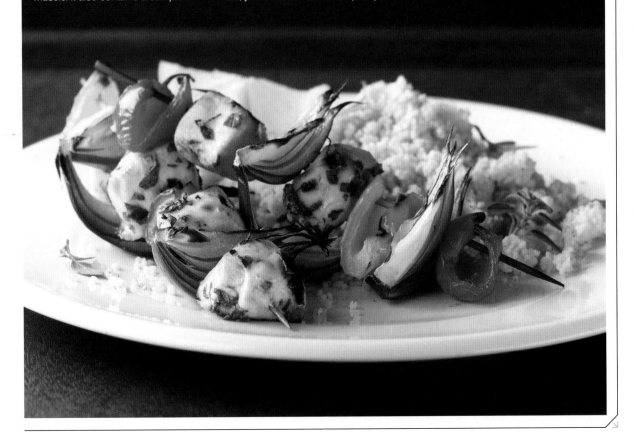

Nutrition | Rules

The rules of eating for muscle

Building muscle is as much about what you do in the kitchen as in the gym. Here's how to get it right

■ The protein myth

Taking on protein is a vital part of muscle-building nutrition but simply scoffing steaks all day won't give you the results you want. In fact, it could have the opposite effect and make you tubbier. That's because the body isn't able to store excess protein, so any that doesn't get used to build muscle either gets used as fuel or turns to fat.

Protein is a necessity for adding muscle, but you don't need any more than 1.5-1.7g of protein per kilo of bodyweight each day to cater for your muscle-building needs. This protein intake should be spread evenly throughout the day to maximise absorption and minimise weight gain. And most should come in the form of complete proteins (food that contains the nine essential amino acids that your body can't produce on it's own), such as meat, fish, milk, eggs and dairy products. This high-quality protein will provide you with all the essential amino acids that are vital for muscles to repair themselves and grow.

■ Calories and carbs

There's a simple equation you need to remember when it comes to building muscle: you have to take in more calories each day than you burn off through activity. But how many more? An average man needs around 2,500 calories a day, but if you want to add muscle that number needs to rise to around 3,000 (as shown in the meal plan overleaf), which will be enough to add muscle without too many excess calories turning into fat.

Of those 3,000 calories, around 60 per cent should come from carbohydrates. The main fuel your body uses when lifting weights is muscle glycogen (stored carbohydrates). If you don't have enough of this, your body will use your muscles to fuel your workout, also known as muscle breakdown. Carb calories increase your chances of gaining pure muscle, not fat.

Make sure you eat a carb-based snack about two hours before training, such as a chicken sandwich made with wholemeal bread. You'll also need to refuel afterwards. Your muscles are at their most responsive immediately after a workout, so eat a snack that has 1g of fast-acting carbohydrate per kilo of bodyweight and is three parts carb to one part protein. This will kick-start an insulin release, which in turn increases the glucose intake in your muscles and stimulates glycogen-making enzymes. A bagel spread with peanut butter and a mashed banana is ideal.

■ Don't forget fat

Another common misconception is that you should steer clear of fat wherever possible. The trick is to avoid bad fats found in greasy fry-ups and opt instead for good ones found in fish, nuts and oils. These should make up 15-30 per cent of your calories and will help to prevent your body from dipping into your precious glycogen stores. They are also essential for the body to absorb fat-soluble vitamins. Evidence suggests that men who don't get enough fatty acids can suffer from low levels of testosterone, the male hormone needed to build bulk. The omega 3 fatty acids also help the body to store glucose as muscle glycogen.

■ Drink, drink and drink

Water, that is. If you're dehydrated your body simply won't work efficiently and that means you won't be able to build muscle. You need water to transport nutrients to the muscles, so don't scrimp. Aim to drink at least two litres a day and, if you can, three. This will not only support your workouts but also ensure your kidneys work efficiently to process all the protein in your diet.

Above all, remember that the numbers on the bathroom scales should only be going up by about a pound a week. If you're gaining weight faster than that it's more likely to be fat than muscle.

How many meals?

To avoid energy crashes, aim to eat five or six meals a day, every two to three hours. This will encourage glycogen storage and muscle-tissue repair, regulating glucose levels, and discourage overeating at meal times. It will also help you take in enough calories; wolfing down 3,000 calories every day isn't as easy as you think.

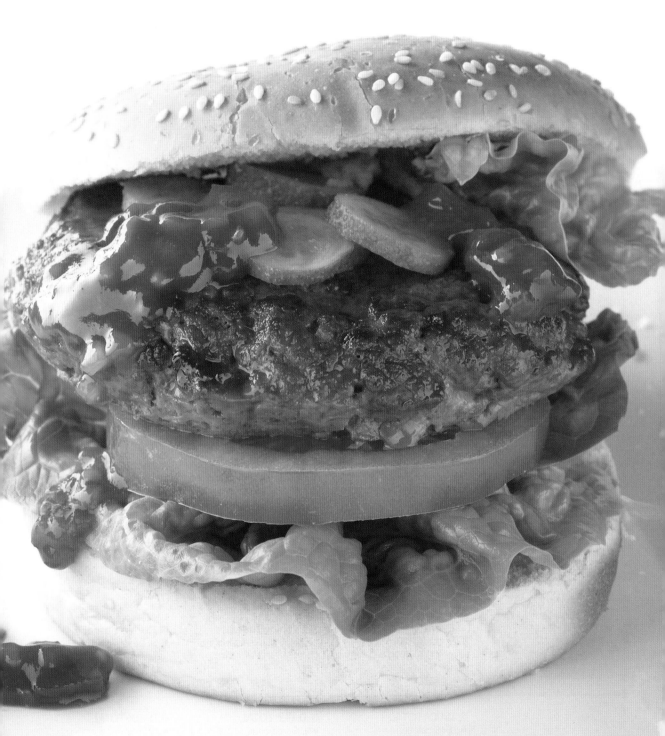

Protein is essential to supply your body with amino acids and should come from meat, fish, eggs and dairy

Nutrition I Meal plan

Muscle meals

This plan contains the kind of foods you should be eating every day to fuel your muscle-building workouts

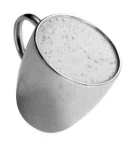

	Monday	**Tuesday**	**Wednesday**

Muscle Tip

Make sure there's a significant amount of protein in the snacks you take before and after weight training sessions to help build and repair muscle.

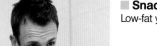

Breakfast
40g muesli with 200ml skimmed milk and 50g fresh berries.
Two slices of wholegrain toast with honey.
Glass of orange juice.

Breakfast
Two poached eggs.
Three slices wholegrain toast with low-fat spread.
Glass of orange juice.

Breakfast
50g porridge oats with 200ml skimmed milk.
Glass of orange juice.

Snack
Low-fat yoghurt and cereal bar.

Snack
Four oatcakes with low-fat cream cheese.
100g fruit berries.

Snack
Muesli bar.
Low-fat fruit yoghurt.
Glass of orange juice.

Lunch
80g salmon baked with 3tbsp cooked basmati rice and steamed veg.

Lunch
Tuna salad with beans, three slices of wholegrain bread and a bowl of mixed salad.

Lunch
Two wholegrain sandwiches with lean meat (four slices of bread) and sprouting bean salad.

Snack
Cereal bar and 100g mixed berries.

Snack
Cereal bar.

Snack
Banana.
Skinny latte and low-fat oat muffin.

Evening meal
125g pasta, 100g grilled chicken, steamed veg, tomato sauce and chickpeas.
Low-fat yoghurt.

Evening meal
Large bowl of seafood chowder with two slices of rye bread.
Fresh fruit salad.

Evening meal
125g pasta with 100g lean turkey Bolognese, steamed veg and a bowl of salad.
Fresh fruit salad.

DAILY TOTAL
- 2,948 calories
- 150g protein
- 542g carbs

DAILY TOTAL
- 2,953 calories
- 119g protein
- 690g carbs

DAILY TOTAL
- 2,912 calories
- 184g protein
- 493g carbs

Meal plan | Nutrition

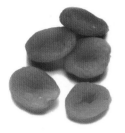
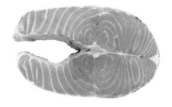
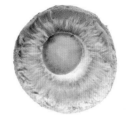
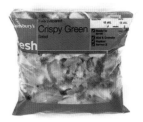

Thursday	Friday	Saturday	Sunday

Breakfast

Thursday: 60g muesli with 200ml skimmed milk and 100g fruit berries. One slice of wholegrain toast with honey. Glass of orange juice.

Friday: 50g porridge oats with 200ml skimmed milk. Glass of orange juice.

Saturday: Two poached eggs. Three slices of wholegrain toast with low-fat spread. Glass of orange juice.

Sunday: Kedgeree. Two slices wholegrain toast with low-fat spread. Glass of orange juice.

Snack

Thursday: Skinny latte and cereal bar.

Friday: Low-fat oat muffin. Glass of orange juice.

Saturday: Skinny latte and cereal bar.

Sunday: Fruit smoothie and cereal bar.

Lunch

Thursday: Bean fajita roll. Low-fat fruit yoghurt and handful dried apricots.

Friday: Three slices of wholegrain toast with low-fat spread. Banana.

Saturday: Lean meat sandwich, fruit salad and low-fat yoghurt.

Sunday: 150g grilled chicken with steamed veg and new potatoes.

Snack

Thursday: Two cereal bars.

Friday: Mixed berries and cereal bar.

Saturday: Three oatcakes with low-fat cream cheese.

Sunday: Two crumpets with peanut butter.

Evening meal

Thursday: 125g lean meat grilled with 3tbsp cooked basmati rice and steamed veg. Fruit salad, low-fat ice cream.

Friday: Salmon with pak choi and steamed veg. Fruit crumble, low-fat ice cream.

Saturday: 100g mushroom risotto with mixed salad. Fresh fruit salad, low-fat ice cream.

Sunday: Thai stir-fried squid with 80g rice noodles. Fresh fruit salad.

DAILY TOTAL

Thursday:
- 3,003 calories
- 124g protein
- 589g carbs

Friday:
- 2,833 calories
- 124g protein
- 479g carbs

Saturday:
- 3,050 calories
- 126g protein
- 562g carbs

Sunday:
- 2,479 calories
- 147g protein
- 366g carbs

Nutrition | Supplements

Supplements explained

Do you or don't you need nutritional supplements? We help you decide

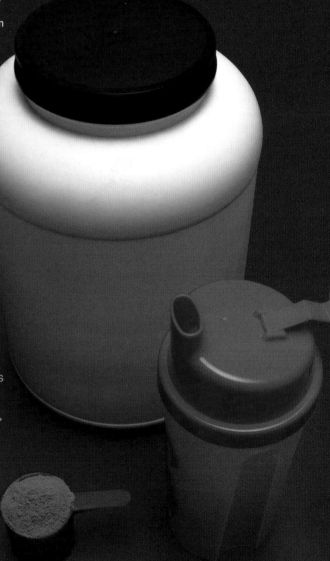

The subject of sports supplements can be confusing. For a start, there's a bewildering array of powders, pills and drinks that all claim to do different things. Some products help you gain weight, some help you lose weight while others help you to perform better at sport. And to make things more difficult, they all seem to contain ingredients you've never heard of. So how do you know what's right for you? And should you even be taking them at all?

Before you decide whether you want to use sports supplements, it's important to realise that supplements aren't magic potions. You can't just glug protein shakes, sit on your sofa and expect to pack on muscle. In order for any supplement to be effective, you need to choose one that suits your workout goal and use it in appropriate quantities alongside a structured and progressive training regime.

What's the point of supplements?
Sports supplements should simply be seen as 'safety nets' to ensure that the body is receiving the nutrients it needs to perform at its best and achieve the look you want. If you are trying to increase muscle mass you know you need to pack away a lot of calories and get the right combination of carbs and amino acids at the best time for muscle replenishment. It is possible to get all this from food – a chicken and rice salad for example – but in today's society where time is short, it is sometimes easier and more convenient to neck a protein shake.

Are they safe?
Yes, when used properly. Before you take any supplement it is a good idea to research the product and stick to a reputable manufacturer – they are usually full of knowledge and willing to give you lots of advice. You should also make sure you follow the dosage on the label. Too much creatine, for example, can be toxic to the kidneys and liver and too much protein will simply turn to lard.

What kind of supplements should I take?
Although there are a lot of supplements to choose from, most fall into one of four categories: muscle builders, fat burners and energy providers. Then you have the various vitamin, mineral and antioxidant supplements that can be valuable to people in serious training. The main categories of supplement are outlined on the opposite page.

The main types of supplement

Whey protein
This is the quickest and most effective protein for muscle recovery and repair after exercise. Weight training increases your need for protein. If you don't get enough you can lose muscle tissue, take longer to recover and your body may break down it's own muscle to use it as energy.

Creatine
There's strong scientific evidence to suggest that creatine can improve muscle strength, power and size. Creatine is produced naturally in the body from three amino acids (proteins). It's found in meat and fish, for example, but not in sufficient quantities to boost muscle building on it's own, which is why you need a supplement.

Fat burners
Known as thermogenics, these are blends of herbs and stimulants that slightly increase body temperature, which can help you burn more calories during exercise. They can be helpful for maintaining energy levels on a low calorie diet. However, regular training and a healthy diet can also boost your metabolosm so their use is questionable.

Energy providers
Usually in the form of drinks, bars and gels, these are good if you want to get that little extra edge when training or if you are looking to train a bit longer than usual. These are pure cabs, which can delay fatigue and improve endurance.

Amino acids
These will help the body release the human growth hormone, which helps prevent the breakdown of muscle tissue during exercise and improve recovery.

Antioxidants
Antioxidants help your body's natural defence against illness by eliminating free radicals, which destroy cells and create oxidative damage. Free radicals are created by intense exercise such as weight training.

Casein
This protein takes seven to eight hours to digest, so it's best taken half an hour before you go to bed. Like whey protein, it helps to repair and build muscle, but it is absorbed more thoroughly so it's highly effective.

Rehydrators
These are usually isotonic sports drinks that will give your body the right blend of sugars and salts during exercise. The blend of water, fast acting carbohydrates and electrolytes will help replenish fluids more efficiently than water alone.

Problem solvers
If you're experiencing diet-related workout problems, these supplements could help

Multivitamins
These are a good option if you're struggling to get the vitamins and minerals you need from your normal diet. Ideally though, you should try to have a nutritious and varied enough diet so that you don't need the help of a multivitamin.

Zinc
Inadequate levels of zinc can hamper muscle growth and weaken your immune system. Regular exercisers need more zinc than inactive people because they need to replenish their red blood cell count and help metabolise fatty acid caused by exercise.

Magnesium
This mineral is essential for burning glucose for fuel and is important for muscle contraction. It's lost in sweat, which is why you may need a supplement if you exercise regularly.

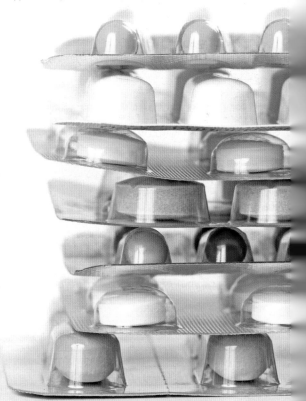

Eating for muscle

Use these nuggets of nutritional advice to make the most of your training

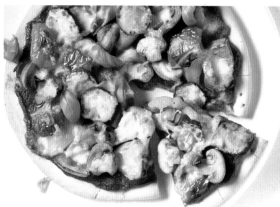

1 Treat yourself

Once you've got the hang of eating nutritionally balanced meals and exercising regularly, you can introduce some treats occasionally. Just make sure your regular meals are healthy and then plan your 'cheat meals' so you can eat whatever you like and enjoy it. By allowing yourself the occasional pizza or bowl of ice cream, you'll satisfy your cravings and have something to look forward to.

2 Eat little and often

The most effective way to sustain even energy levels across the day is to spread your calories over five or six small meals, rather than three big ones. By eating lots of small meals you'll keep your metabolism burning and your blood sugar levels stable. Eating regularly also prevents fat storage, keeps hunger at bay and provides better support for muscle recovery.

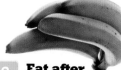

3 Eat after exercise

Weight training seriously depletes your body's energy supplies, so you'll need to get some fast-acting carbs inside you, along with quality protein to fuel and repair muscles. Your body is also most responsive to food straight after training so eat a snack such as a banana and peanut butter sandwich or a bagel with cream cheese and sliced tomato within 30 minutes of finishing your session.

4 Always have breakfast

Skipping breakfast may seem like a good way of losing the fat that's hiding your muscles but it isn't – studies have found that people who ate breakfast were less likely to be overweight than those who skipped it. A breakfast based around complex carbs and protein helps cut cravings for sweet or starchy foods, as well as boosting the metabolism. Good breakfast foods include wholegrain cereals, porridge, eggs on wholemeal toast and fruit.

5 Cut down on booze

They don't call it a beer belly for nothing. The average pint of lager contains almost 200 'empty' calories, and when calories don't have any use they are usually stored as fat. If you're serious about training, keep your sessions in the pub to a minimum.

6 Get your five a day

Your body needs to be well stocked with vitamins and minerals to keep energy levels up and boost your immune system. Fruits and vegetables are also extremely filling thanks to their high volume of water. This allows you to fill up with fewer calories and get enough fat-absorbing fibre.

7 Have a protein snack at bedtime

Have some cottage cheese or a low-fat yogurt before you hit the hay. They are full of slow-acting protein, which will help regenerate your muscles while you sleep.

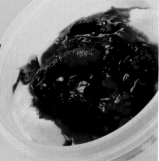

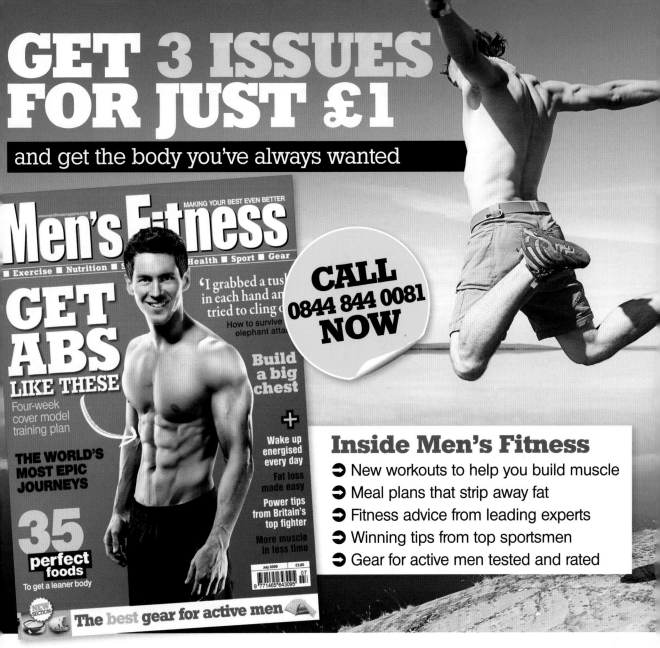

GET 3 ISSUES FOR JUST £1

and get the body you've always wanted

CALL 0844 844 0081 NOW

Inside Men's Fitness

➔ New workouts to help you build muscle
➔ Meal plans that strip away fat
➔ Fitness advice from leading experts
➔ Winning tips from top sportsmen
➔ Gear for active men tested and rated

Claim 3 issues of *Men's Fitness* today for £1 and start getting results

Order online today at
www.dennismags.co.uk/mensfitness or
CALL 0844 844 0081
using offer code G0906HWG

If during **your 3 trial issues**, you decide *Men's Fitness* isn't for you, simply cancel and you won't pay a penny more. Best of all, if you continue reading you'll **SAVE 12%** on the shop price, and pay just £19.95 every 6 issues

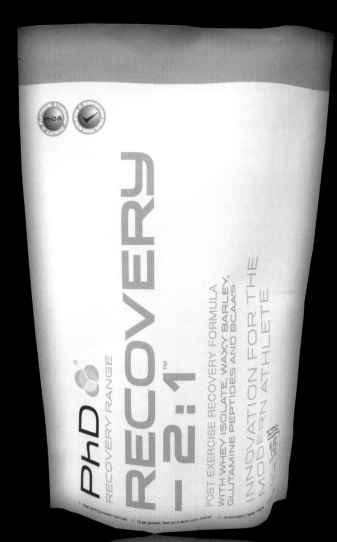
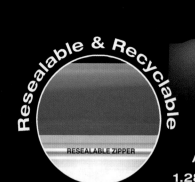